Heat and Human Interaction

By Bhargav Dave and Jerrold Petrofsky

Printed in the United States of America

First Printing, Sep 22, 2016

E-Book ISBN 978-0-9981743-0-3

Print Book ISBN 978-0-9981743-1-0

Srinivas University Press

2804 Field Hollow Dr,
Pearland, Texas, USA 77584

FOREWORD

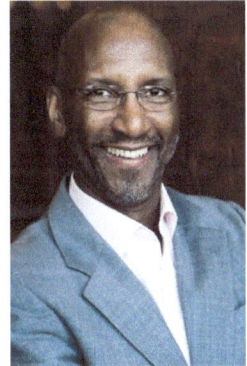

Dr. Craig Jackson

Skin is the largest organ of the body and performs a vast number of functions; it serves as our protection from the elements, regulates body temperature, and allows us to experience sensation, both pleasant and unpleasant. But more than that, the skin is often the first thing people notice when they meet us, and it has a tremendous impact on one's psychological status. Just turn on the television and you will see that every other commercial is about medication for psoriasis, rosacea, eczema or acne. In many ways, the skin is both the gateway and the gatekeeper of our physical experience.

This book, which provides a comprehensive study of heat and its valuable role in treatment modalities, focuses on the skin's vital role in our overall health. It covers every aspect of the skin, beginning with the basic anatomy of the skin (i.e. the intricacies of thermoregulation and the thermo-receptors and the effect of dry heat and moist heat on the body) and the interplay between it and the other systems of the body (i.e. warning us of danger through sensory pain). This manuscript also explains the various injuries and diseases affecting the skin, such as coagulative necrosis of the skin and acute inflammation to infections and malignancies. More importantly, it explores the various treatment modalities, including those under the umbrella of ThermoTherapy, which utilizes heat in physical therapy. Building on a foundation of thermo-mechanics, or the underlying science of heat transfer, burns and physiology, the authors provide a comprehensive understanding of cutting edge treatment that focuses on effectively treating the patient while maximizing comfort and care.

Since the days of Hippocrates, the greatest challenge for any healthcare provider has been to balance scientific knowledge with empathy for the patient, to treat man as a whole unit. This book, with its dual focus on understanding complex systems of the body and delivering compassionate care, provides an excellent roadmap in that regard. Bhargav Dave, whom I had the pleasure of meeting in 2011 when I presented him with his Post-Professional Masters of Physical Therapy degree from School of Allied Health Professions has demonstrated a thorough understanding of the mechanics of physical therapy, as well as his commitment to those the patients he serves. This book is an invaluable resource for others also pursuing a career as physical therapists.

Dr. Craig Jackson

Dean,
School of Allied Health Professions
Loma Linda University

PREFACE

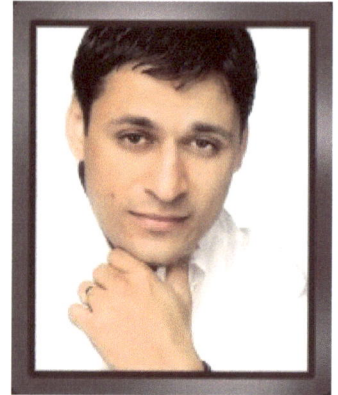

Manish Patel

I feel honored to be part of this very unique book from such a young dynamic and divine writer Dr. Bhargav Dave. Dr. Dave has not written this book from his mind, but his deeper part of consciousness. Like one ray of white light enters prism and exit as seven colors, giving birth to duality, if we all look beyond these seven colors we can look at its source and feel oneness with one another. One must silent his mind to be able to access deeper part of his consciousness. When any information comes from this deeper, invisible part, it becomes scripture. I am sure this book will serve as a scientific scripture for generations to come. We are standing at a cross road in the history where the world needs more of such scientific scriptures. I know Bhargav for a long time and I am sure his consciousness has touched the other side of the prism. He is very compassionate towards humanity. I know a very few people who has achieved this height at such a young age. He has won International significant achievement award (under 30 year's category) for his scientific advancements and his work in the area of health science field. He has published several papers in international journals and served on editorial advisory committee and peer reviewer for several international journals. He is the chosen one by the divine to awaken the frozen ones. This book will definitely serve its purpose and touch you at your core.

Thank you Bhargav for providing me with this very unique opportunity to write a few words about this book where heat has been explained like never before.

May god bless us all.
Thank you.

Manish Patel

Author, Second Childhood
President,
Manish Therapy Services

4

MEET AUTHORS

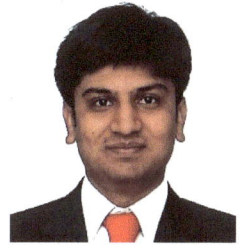

Dr. Bhargav Dave

Dr. Bhargav Dave, PT, DPT is an Inventor, Physical Therapist and Researcher in field of Health Sciences. He has published several high quality research articles in high ranking international journals. He has won International Significant Achievement Award in under 30 year's category for his unique contribution in the field of health science. He is also winner of C.P. Nair Oration Award from Indian Association of Physiotherapists. Dr. Dave was also nominated for Hamilton Youth Council Award for outstanding community work in Hamilton, New Zealand. He has been featured several times on several radio shows, Times of India, Divya Bhaskar, Houston Chronicle and Sandesh news papers for his research work.

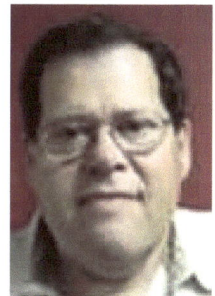

Dr. Jerrold Petrofsky

Dr. Jerrold Petrofsky is an inventor, a professor and a renowned research scientist with international fame. He was nominated for Nobel Prize in Medicine. He holds a Ph. D. in Neurophysiology from Saint Louis University. He also holds Honorary Ph. D. from Pennsylvania State University. He also has a JD from Western State University. He was director at Physical Fitness Laboratory at Loma Linda University. He has been awarded with Congressional Recognition Certificate by U.S. Congress. He has countless awards and qualifications. He has published 550+ research papers in international journals and, He has presented over 115 papers in conference. He also holds patents to 31+ devices/techniques.

ACKOWLEDGEMENTS

I would like to thank my wife Asmi Dave for helping me, inspiring me every step of the way in making this book a reality. I would like to thank my parents for giving me their best and shaping me in a better human being. I would like to thank my daughter Myra for loving me unconditionally and filling my life with joy and hope. I would like to dedicate this book to my mentor and guru Manish Patel and my wife Asmi Dave on their birthday Sep 22, 2016. You have seen me going through all the phases of this book. Lastly, I would like to thank the Divine Mother and Sri Aurobindo for making possible the impossible.

I would like to thank PRO and Professor Dr. Ajay Kumar of Srinivas University (School of Physical Therapy) and Dr. Rajasekar, Principal, Srinivas University (School of Physical Therapy) for their guidance and continuous support.

Table of Contents

CHAPTER 1

The Anatomy of Skin

Bhargav Dave, PT, DPT

Learning Objectives:

1. Layers of skin,
2. Physiology of skin,
3. Thermoregulation,
4. Different skin receptors and its functions.

The Segumentum Commune, or skin, is the largest organ of the body. It protects our internal organs from the external environment (i.e. microorganisms, air with dust particles and external mechanical injuries); it also plays a vital role in perceiving that environment (through sensory nerves) and in the process of thermoregulation. To some extent, it also plays a role in excretion and absorption. The thickness of the skin varies depending upon gender and age; male skin is much thicker than female skin, and the skin of children is relatively thin and becomes thicker as one gets older. However, between the ages of forty and fifty the skin begins to grow thinner again as it gradually loses elastic fibers and appendages.

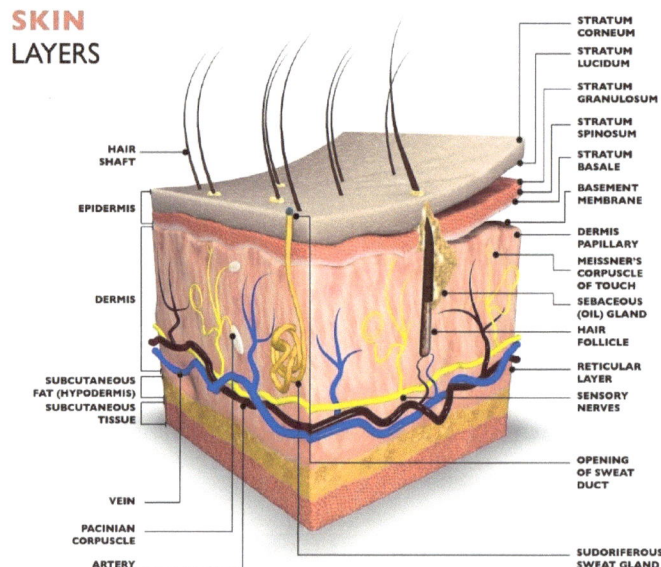

Diagram 1: Layers of the skin

- **Layers of Skin:**

The vascular layer, or corium, is made up of connective tissue. It contains vascular papillae on its surface and has sebaceous glands and hair follicles under it. The outer layer is covered by a layer of stratified epithelium called the epidermis and has four layers, from within outward as follows: (a) stratum mucosum, (b) stratum granulosum, (c) stratum lucidum, and (d) stratum corneum. The stratum mucosum is also made of many layers of cells, which are connected with tiny fibrils making bridges, which again have intercellular clefts for the exchange of lymph (Guyton, 2008). The stratum granulosum also contains two or three layers of cells, all of which contain an eleidin substance, an intermediate substance in the formation of keratin. These cells are in a transitional stage between the protoplasmic cells of the stratum mucosum and the stratum germinativum, or basal layer and are superficial to the dermo-epidermal junction. This basal layer is attached to the basement membrane via hemidesmosomes (Guyton, 2008).

The epidermis differs in thickness in some areas, such as the palms and soles. The outer two layers are the stratum corneum and stratum mucosum (deeper layers of the cells). The epidermis consists of linear furrows dividing the outer body surface area into different shapes that correspond to the folds created by movement; for example, the epidermal ridges that are visible on the palms and soles and help create resistance between the palm or sole and an object's surface (Guyton, 2008). The epidermis has no blood vessels and is entirely dependent on the underlying dermis for nutrients and disposal of waste. The process disposal of waste happens at the dermo-epidermal junction. The epidermis is composed of stratified epithelium, which is primarily made of keratinocytes from the deeper dermis to the superficial epidermis (Griffiths, Barker, Bleiker, Chalmers, & Creamer, 2016).

The division and differentiation of keratinocytes move from the deep to the superficial layer. Upon reaching the stratum corneum, they can be identified as keratinocytes and are shed during epidermal turnover. The stratum corneum makes up most of the epidermis due to its large size and presence. They make a fifteen to one-hundred-cell-thick layer, depending on the anatomical region, which also offers protection against environmental elements (Guyton, 2008).

Keratinocytes form a tight-knit epithelium at the surface of the skin, which protects the body from the external environment. The formation and maintenance of the epidermis are maintained by the processes of cell proliferation, differentiation, and self-renewal (Romano & Sinha, 2011)

The stratum lucidum consists of cells with a substance called keratohyalin. The stratum corneum, the deepest of all the above layers, is referred to as a "horny layer" because it contains the horny material called keratin. The cells of the stratum corneum are the largest in the epidermis (Guyton, 2008).

The epidermis houses the pigment melanin, which determines the skin color. This is mainly contained in the layers of stratum mucosum, and gradually disappears in the superficial layers. Langerhans cells, produced from the bone marrow, are present in the basal layer and the granular layers of the epidermis and act as antigen-presenting cells. They ingest foreign particles, cut them into small peptide fragments, bind them with histo compatible complexes and present them to lymphocytes. This causes activation of the immune system (Romano & Sinha, 2011). Contact hypersensitivity is an example of activation of this component of the immune system. The epidermis thus helps protect the inner layers of the skin that contain nerves and vessels. Langerhans cells are absent in stratum corneum layer of the epidermis but maintain a prominent presence in stratum spinosm layer (Romano & Sinha, 2011).

The corium, or true skin, is a variably thick and flexible skin called the dermis. It is a complex structure consisting of two layers: the papillary dermis, which is the superficial layer, and the deeper reticular dermis. The papillary dermis is thin and made up of loose connective tissue that contains capillaries, elastic fibers, reticular fibers, and some collagen (Romano & Sinha, 2011). The reticular dermis, which is composed of dense connective tissue, contains large blood vessels, elastic fibers, and collagen fibers arranged in parallel layers. The dermis is thicker on the palms and soles (the lateral rather than medial areas) and on posterior surfaces of the body, and thinner on genital surfaces (i.e. the scrotum and penis), as well as on the eyelids, where the skin is very delicate (Griffiths, Barker, Bleiker, Chalmers, & Creamer, 2016). The dermis also contains fibroblasts, elastic connective tissue, blood vessels, nerve endings, lymphatics vessels, mast cells and epidermal appendages (Griffiths, Barker, Bleiker, Chalmers, & Creamer, 2016).

The dermis is surrounded by a gel-like substance comprised of mucopolysaccharides, chondroitin sulfates, and glycoproteins. The layer of the dermis is irregular and covers the adipose tissue, also known as subcutaneous fat. The papillary layer has vascular papillae, which are perpendicular and very minute. They are larger in the areas such as palms and soles, forming ridges (Romano & Sinha, 2011). Between the papillae are ducts of the sudoriferous glands that open at the ridges. Papillae contain fibrillated tissues, and have few elastic fibers, capillary loops, and tactile corpuscles. The dermal papillae of the dermis contain capillaries and lymphatic capillaries and are perpendicular to the skin's surface (Griffiths, Barker, Bleiker, Chalmers, & Creamer, 2016). They are surrounded by projections of the epidermis that increase the surface area. This contributes to the exchange of oxygen, nutrients and waste products between the dermis and the epidermis (Griffiths, Barker, Bleiker, Chalmers, & Creamer, 2016).

The dermo-epidermal junction is a basement membrane connecting the dermis to the epidermis. It is made up of two laters: the lamina lucida, a thin layer just below the basal layer of the epidermis, and the lamina densa, a thick layer in direct contact with the dermis (Guyton, 2008). So the deepest cutaneous wounds also can re-epithealise with these cells. Epidermal appendages are intra-dermal and are aligned with the epithelial cells. They can divide and are seen in differentiation. Different appendages are hair, nails, sebaceous glands, sweat glands, mammary glands and apocrine glands (Griffiths, Barker, Bleiker, Chalmers, & Creamer, 2016). These are derived from skin cells. In cases of the destruction of the epidermis (such as superficial burns or other traumas, abrasions and skin-graft harvesting), skin appendages act as a source of epithelial cells and help in re-epithelialisation for healing (Guyton, 2008).

Hair is present almost everywhere on the skin, the exceptions beingthe palms and soles and the inner surfaces of the labia, prepuce, and the penis glans (Guyton, 2008). Hair contains a root and a shaft and is attached to the skin through a structure called a hair bulb, which is lodged in a hair follicle. There is a sebaceous gland at the hair follicle, and the bottom of the hair follicle lie papillae (Griffiths, Barker, Bleiker, Chalmers, & Creamer, 2016). They exist continuously with the dermis. Sebaceous glands produce sebum, oil produced from the breakdown of triglycerides and fatty acids, giving wax esters, squalene, cholesterol esters, and cholesterol. Sebum, in conjunction with the hair follicle, helps to lubricate the skin, thus protecting it against friction, and also makes it less permeable to moisture. The hair follicle consists of two layers, the dermic and the epidermic coats. The dermic layer is very vascular and contains nervous tissue. The hair bulb, which is composed of epithelial cells, is what gives hair its pigment. The hair shaft has three parts: medulla, cortex, and cuticle. Each hair follicle goes through a growth cycle with three main phases: anagen, catagen, and telogen (Griffiths, Barker, Bleiker, Chalmers, & Creamer, 2016).

The anagen phase is a long stage (three to five years) that produces growth; the catagen phase is significantly shorter (two to three weeks) and is a transitional phase, and the telogen phase causes shedding of the hair (Griffiths, Barker, Bleiker, Chalmers, & Creamer, 2016). At any given time, follicles can be found in all three stages of hair growth on various areas of the body. This is important to note with regard to laser hair removal, as follicles in the anagen phase are more prone to destruction than resting follicles, which are more resistant (Griffiths, Barker, Bleiker, Chalmers, & Creamer, 2016). This explains why multiple treatments of a given area may be necessary to ensure lasting results. Sebaceous glands, also called holocrine glands, are present on the entire surface of the body except the palms, soles, and dorsum of the feet. As mentioned above, sebaceous glands aid in the production and secretion of sebum; these glands are the largest and highest in number on the face and scalp, which make those regions more susceptible to acne vulgaris (Griffiths, Barker, Bleiker, Chalmers, & Creamer, 2016).

Sweat glands, also called eccrine glands, are also present throughout the body, with the exception of the vermillion border of the lips, the external ear canal, penis glans, nail beds and labia minora. They are highest in number on the palms, soles, and axillae (Guyton, 2008). Sweat glands produce sweat to cool the body through the process of evaporation. Sweat gland activity is controlled by the hypothalamus through innervations via sympathetic nerve fibers (Guyton, 2008). Sweat excretion is stimulated when the core body temperature exceeds a certain point. The apocrine and mammary glands are similar to sweat glands, and are present in axillae, the anogenital region, in the breasts (mammary glands), the external ear canal and modified in the margin of the eyelid (Moll's glands) (Griffiths, Barker, Bleiker, Chalmers, & Creamer, 2016). These glands produce a distinct smell and become active only during puberty and as such are considered vestigial structures. The mammary gland is a type of apocrine gland, modified to perform a highly specialized function (Griffiths, Barker, Bleiker, Chalmers, & Creamer, 2016).

Cutaneous vessels originate from the source arteries, or muscular vessels. Each source vessel supplies a vascular area from bone to skin, which is called an angiosome (Griffiths, Barker, Bleiker, Chalmers, & Creamer, 2016). These cutaneous vessels go through the connective tissue framework and provide blood/nutrients to the tissues that come in close contact with bone, muscle, fascia, nerve, and fat (Griffiths, Barker, Bleiker, Chalmers, & Creamer, 2016). The dermis has horizontal arrangements of superficial and deep plexuses. Cutaneous vessels forms anastomose with other dermal vessels to form a continuous network in the skin. This parallel network of vessels helps in random skin flap survival (Griffiths, Barker, Bleiker, Chalmers, & Creamer, 2016).

Thermoregulation means that skin has a natural heat conductivity that causes heat loss due to the evaporation of sweat, or convection, that occurs in cutaneous vessels (Griffiths, Barker, Bleiker, Chalmers, & Creamer, 2016). Cutaneous blood is oxygen rich, needed for metabolism. Thus, an enormous amount of heat can be exchanged via the regulation of the cutaneous blood flow (Griffiths, Barker, Bleiker, Chalmers, & Creamer, 2016). The hypothalamus acts as a thermoregulatory center that controls the sympathetic nervous system for vasoconstriction and vasodilatation of cutaneous vessels (Griffiths, Barker, Bleiker, Chalmers, & Creamer, 2016).

The type of skin plays a vital role in thermoregulation, the type of the skin plays a vital role. For non-hairy skin, the heat loss is insensible (Guyton, 2008). This kind of skin is present over palms and soles, towards the distal end of the body. It has a larger blood supply, arteriovenous anastomoses and a large surface-to-volume ratio (Guyton, 2008). Thus, heat is transferred quickly to the environment as the flow of blood is increased. For example, the flow of blood in a finger can increase by five times when necessary (Guyton, 2008).

Skin lymphatics play a role in the conservation of plasma proteins; they remove foreign material, antigenic substances, and bacteria. The lymphatic capillaries are unvalved (Griffiths, Barker, Bleiker, Chalmers, & Creamer, 2016). The superficial dermal vessels drain in the deep dermal and subdermal vessels. They form a large lymphatic channel, which passes through the lymph nodes on their way to join the venous circulation (Griffiths, Barker, Bleiker, Chalmers, & Creamer, 2016).

- **Skin Innervations**

It is incredibly important to be able to discern the sense of pressure, extremes of temperature, and trauma (pain), and there are various structures present in the skin to detect these stimuli. Merkel cells and Meissner corpuscles, which are found in the dermal papillae and are highest in number at the fingertips, perceive a light touch. Pacini corpuscles are present deep in the dermis discern pressure (Griffiths, Barker, Bleiker, Chalmers, & Creamer, 2016).

Pain passes through the afferent free nerve endings found in the basal layer of the epidermis. Krause bulbs and Ruffini corpuscles detect cold and heat, respectively. Heat, cold, and proprioception are sensed in the superficial dermis also. Cutaneous nerves are similar to those of blood vessels of the skin. The area supplied by a single spinal nerve is termed a dermatome. Adjacent dermatomes may overlap, which is important to allow us to identify pain sites (Griffiths, Barker, Bleiker, Chalmers, & Creamer, 2016).

The skin phototype determines a person's skin color and is dependent upon the amount of melanin pigment present in the skin. Pigmentation is usually inherited, but can also be the result of disease or hormonal changes during pregnancy. Regardless of the cause, it is important to note variances in pigmentation when giving treatment with ultraviolet radiation, for it can cause adverse effects such as burns and skin tanning in a particular skin type and color (Griffiths, Barker, Bleiker, Chalmers, & Creamer, 2016).

When observed under a microscope, the structure of the skin is almost the same in every individual. That said, there are external differences, mostly in the epidermis. For example, while the stratum corneum is more compact in dark skin than light skin, it is equal in thickness regardless of pigmentation. In addition, twenty cell layers are seen in dark skin as compared with just sixteen layers present in light skin. Darker skin also has more lipids in the epidermis than light skin; thus, there is a greater cellular cohesion, causing difficulty in stripping off the dark layer. It also indicates comparatively less permeability of dark skin to certain substances (Griffiths, Barker, Bleiker, Chalmers, & Creamer, 2016).

Finally, the epidermis of dark skin is also less hydrated than that of light skin, which results in greater electrical resistance. And, while dark skin and light skin have the same number of sweat glands, they are affected differently by changes in climate; for example, the dark-skinned individuals should sustain the moist heat better, and the light-skinned individuals should sustain dry heat better (Griffiths, Barker, Bleiker, Chalmers, & Creamer, 2016).

Our skin is exposed to a constant barrage of stimuli in our external environment. Sensory receptors present in the dermis and superficial muscles act as a direct interface between those stimuli and the body. Regulation of body temperature if a key function of these sensors; heat receptors in the dermis detect the temperature outside the body and make changes to the temperature inside the body to adjust to the external environment (Nicol, 2005).

The thermo-receptor is a type of sensory receptor or neuron that has free nerve endings and plays a significant role in perceiving a change in temperature. These thermo-receptors are unmyelinated C-fibers, which are part of the peripheral nervous system, and sense a maximum temperature of 45 degrees C° and minimum of 30 degrees C°(Nicol, 2005). They have a low velocity of conduction. The stimulus for these types of the receptor is of course heat, which causes an increase in the rate of activity potential. The reverse is true in cold receptors, where the action-potential rate increases with the cold and decreases with the heat (Nicol, 2005).

A subtype of these thermoreceptors is the nociceptive fibers, which sense painful, noxious heat sensations. In addition to free nerve endings, thermos-receptors also have Krause end bulbs, which act as cold receptors, and Ruffini endings, which act as heat receptors (Nicol, 2005). Krause end bulbs have oval bodies, with a capsule of connective tissues. They are the part of epineurium of the nerves. The Ruffini endings are large dendrites with elongated, spindle-shaped capsules contained by the deep layers of the skin (Nicol, 2005).

Thus, with deep tissue burn, they get burned, and the person does not experience pain (due to damage to the nerve ending and nerve carrying signal itself). They respond over an extended period of heating, and their adaptation is minimal. These thermoreceptors are less sensitive to absolute temperature but very sensitive to any change in temperature, so a person feels the change in temperature when both the hot and cold receptor gets stimulated concurrently (Nicol, 2005).

The mechanism for sensing heat and the course of the Lissauer's tract is where any change in temperature is received by the sensory heat receptors, and it is passed through the spinal cord through the Lissauer's tract (Griffiths, Barker, Bleiker, Chalmers, & Creamer, 2016). This tract synapses with the neurons of the dorsal horn in its grey matter; these are the second-order neurons. The axons from these neurons decussate and enter the spinothalamic tract, to the thalamus (Nicol, 2005).

- **Thermoregulation and thermoreception**

Thermoregulation is largely controlled by the hypothalamus, a gland in the brain often referred to as the "thermostat of the body". When the thermo-receptors sense a change in the temperature outside, they signal the hypothalamus which in turn gives the signal for vasoconstriction, thereby preventing the loss of excess heat from the body. In contrast, when the body experiences excess heat the hypothalamus sends a signal for dilatation of blood vessels, which supplies more blood to the outer part of the skin. Thus, the body loses excess heat and causes regulation of body temperature. In this process, the hair muscles relax to cool the body in a time of excess heat, and they constrict in excess cold, and so the hair stands erect (Griffiths, Barker, Bleiker, Chalmers, & Creamer, 2016).

The pathway of thermoreception begins withthe thermoreceptors. Changes in temperature pass through the spinal cord and on to the thalamus, leading to the brain's somatosensory cortex. Any heat sensation that becomes too high is felt as pain because pain and temperature share the same tract for carrying the sensation (Nicol, 2005). Cutaneous receptors such as Merkel disks and Meisner corpuscles are present in the skin, giving the tactile senses of hot and cold temperatures and pressure. Some areas of the skin sense hot or cold sensations, some sense pain, and others sense pressure. Pain receptors are the most numerous, but all are present in every area of the skin, which is why any area of the body can feel pain, et cetera (Griffiths, Barker, Bleiker, Chalmers, & Creamer, 2016). That's because the sensory systems work with a few of the sensory fibers decussating to the other side of the tract and then reach the thalamus. Should there be any damage to the tracts, only that particular sensation gets affected while others are still felt as usual (Griffiths, Barker, Bleiker, Chalmers, & Creamer, 2016).

Cold receptors are present in greater numbers than hot receptors. They sense the temperature as well as any change in the temperature (Stoll, 1977). Pain is transmitted through A-delta fibers, which are myelinated and conduct pain quickly, and through C-delta fibers, which are non-myelinated and conduct pain slowly (Bigley, 1990). The pathway for pain perception goes through these pain receptors via the sensory nerves carrying the pain to dorsal root ganglions through the sensory nerves. These nerve fibers pass through the lateral column of the spinal cord tract, then through the Lissauer's tract, progressing further to the substantia gelatinosa to the third-degree neuron in the thalamus. The areas that perceive pain sensations in the cortex are the somatosensory areas one and two; the pre- and post-central gyrus (Bigley, 1990). Thus, knowledge of sensory system anatomy can greatly assist the physical therapist in determining the exact reason for the patient's neuropathology, and how to treat it.

CHAPTER 2

The Physiology of Skin

Bhargav Dave, PT, DPT

Learning Objectives:

1. Body temperature,
2. Mechanism behind heat regulation,
3. Heat therapy and pain.

The last chapter discussed the anatomy of the skin and how it interacts with systems of the body to perform its many functions, including but not limited to protection, temperature regulation, vitamin D production, wound healing, homeostasis, and excretion (Bigley, 1990). This chapter will delve more deeply into those functions.

- **Body Temperature**

The sympathetic nervous system is responsible for maintaining ideal body temperature. The human body has the remarkable ability to maintain a constant temperature, between 98°F and 100°F, when the temperature of the surrounding atmosphere is between 68°F and 130°F. Heat transfer from the external environment occurs in the form of radiation, conduction, and convection (Nicol, 2005).

The high temperature in the environment causes skin temperature to rise; excess heat then evaporates from the body in the form of perspiration, thus cooling down the body. If the temperature goes below 37 degrees C°, the body tries to preserve heat in the body and starts producing more heat. The mechanism by which body works to preserve heat includes vasoconstriction, which decreases blood-flow to the skin. Shivering occurs to preserve heat from the muscles (Nicol, 2005).

The amount of heat lost from the skin is directly proportional to the amount of blood-flow to the dermis. This blood-flow is determined by the body, based on ambient temperature. This mechanism is employed to maintain an ideal appropriate temperature between internal body temperature and ambient temperature. Heat has to go through varies structures like the dermis, adipose tissue (or fat) and other subcutaneous tissues. Since the adipose tissue is a poor conductor of heat, it offers some insulation from heat loss (Nicol, 2005).

Extreme temperatures will always result in a difference between the skin and ambient temperature and therefore some heat loss or gain. In extreme cold, skin temperature can only decrease to so much before frostbite sets in. If the body does not warm up, rapid heat loss can occur, leading to hypothermia and eventually death. Think of the body as a heater, attempting to increase ambient temperature. As mentioned above, in an extremely hot climate, perspiration releases excess heat, thereby preventing the body from going into heat stroke (Griffiths, Barker, Bleiker, Chalmers, & Creamer, 2016).

- **Heat Regulation and Physical Therapy**

Superficial heating modalities are extensively used in physical therapy and physical medicine. They work by increasing circulation in the superficial tissues and hence cause healing. However, recent studies suggest that in people who are overweight, certain modalities (i.e. hydro collator packs, whirlpool baths short wave diathermy, and ultrasound) are less effective because of the limited ability of subcutaneous fat to transfer heat. However, other modalities such as hot packs can change the temperature by moving heat to deep muscle, so long as they are applied over a longer period of time (Griffiths, Barker, Bleiker, Chalmers, & Creamer, 2016).

Hyperthermia occurs when there is more heat produced than is dissipated. Also, a significant amount of heat is accumulated because of the metabolic production of heat. Thus, to avoid excess heat accumulation, the body responds by sweating and a change in the cutaneous blood flow. Heat adaptation occurs when there is a rise in temperature in the external environment. This happens after repeated exposure to heat. After this repeated exposure, the body adapts so that the temperature rise is minimal, with less of an increase in heart rate. This is because of increased sweat with a low salt concentration. However, this effect of adaptation remains temporary if the frequency of exposure to heat is reduced. Therefore, heat adaptation is greater in people who live in hot climates, such as tropical regions. That is, an increase in the body temperature and heart rate is comparatively lower than that of individuals who are not long-term residents in such hot areas (Hori, 1995).

Cutaneous circulation during heat transfer occurs when there is an exchange of heat between the internal body and external environment, and depends on the temperature outside and inside the body. It occurs with the evaporation of heat and also through the evaporation of water through sweat, the lungs, and air passages. Another type of non- evaporative heat exchange occurs when the internal temperature increases. This occurs by an increase in blood circulation, that is, cutaneous circulation, causing heat to dissipate (Hori, 1995).

There has been necessary pain sensation research in which the application of heating modalities in treating thermal pain was studied. The mechanism of thermal pain involves an extreme increase or decrease in temperature through a thermo- mechanical method. This thermal pain mechanism was investigated along with the mechanisms of transduction, transmission, modulation and perception, to make the concept of thermal pain relief clear and enhance their application in the complications associated with thermal injuries (Hori, 1995).

Relative heating means the amount of energy being converted to heat at any given location. Thus, the practitioner can select a modality that provides the highest temperature at the affected area without increasing it beyond the tolerance level of the patient. This rise in temperature is dependent on the type of heat, its conductivity, and the duration of the treatment. Thus, the target area temperature, before the application of a modality, decides the rise and distribution of the temperature. There is a clear difference in the allocation of heat between superficial and deep tissue temperature, so the therapist has to select the modality correctly to get the desired result. For this to occur, the heat should be at maximum up to the tolerance of the patient. At the site of the lesion, the rise of temperature should be the maximum necessary to get the maximum effect (Griffiths, Barker, Bleiker, Chalmers, & Creamer, 2016).

When the heat is applied to a painful area, the following physiology occurs due to the heat-sensitive calcium channels. As the amount of heat increases, there is a rise in the intracellular calcium. This stimulates sensory nerves due to the production of the action potential. The channels mentioned above, TRPV1, and TRPV2 receptors are sensitive to noxious heat and another type, TRPV4, is sensitive to physiological heat. When they are activated, they can deactivate the purine pain receptors, which are mediating pain receptors located in the peripheral small nerve endings. Therefore, heat can reduce peripheral pain; when pain comes from deep tissues, heat can stimulate the peripheral pain receptors, which in turn can reduce the deep pain (Nicol, 2005).

Temperature can also affect the exchange of calcium and sodium between neural cells. Upon heating the skin, the temperature of superficial tissues rises and chemical mediators also rises, which leads to the release of histamine and prostaglandins. The physiologic effects of heat application include pain relief and tissue healing. Deep heating reduces the sensitivity of the nerves; there is an increase in metabolism and bloodflow to the area, and a decrease in muscle spindle activity, causing muscle relaxation and a consequent reduction in joint stiffness. Heat stimulates the receptors in the skin. They are connected to the cutaneous blood vessels, which cause the release of bradykinin. Bradykinin relaxes the smooth muscle of the walls of the blood vessels, which also causes vasodilation. The decrease in muscle spindle activity leads to muscle relaxation. The alpha motor neurons and the extra-fusal muscle fiber fire slowly, causing relaxation of muscle and decrease in muscle tone (Nicol, 2005).

It is incumbent upon all physical therapists to become familiar with the sensory system so they can understand how the body receives stimuli and the application of heat therapy can be most effective. The senses of the body connect the external environment with the body. Sensations can be somatic or they can be visceral. Somatic sensations are easily recognized, and are categorized according to their placement in the body and the types of functions they perform. Extroceptive sensations are a variety of sensations present in the skin and mucosal membranes. Tactile sensations are misinterpreted if there is a loss of other sensations. Pain sensations can either become hyper- or hypo- (that is, oversensitive or not perceived at all). Similarly, thermal sensations – those relating to heat sensation -

can be affected, resulting in thermal hyperesthesia or thermalgesia (loss of heat sensation) (Nicol, 2005).

Given the above, the patient must be tested for pain sensation prior to the application of heat therapy. The areas for tactile, temperature, and pain are the same all over the skin. Particular emphasis should be given to the area where the external heat is to be applied. The distal portions, as well as the areas in the center, are checked (Griffiths, Barker, Bleiker, Chalmers, & Creamer, 2016). One side's sensations are compared with the other side. If the areas to be treated have diminished or are hypersensitive to pain, greater care must be taken in the application of thermal heat. To test temperature sensing, an application of ice followed by warm water is applied to the skin. If the temperature is too low -that is, below five degrees or a temperature above 45 degrees – the patient will experience an unpleasant sensation. It is helpful for the patient to close his or her eyes during the testing; this is because identifying the sensation of pain is easier than identifying the stimulus (Griffiths, Barker, Bleiker, Chalmers, & Creamer, 2016).

The therapist also needs to check whether the patient is experiencing any other unpleasant sensation, including numbness. The role of cortical sensations is the identification and discrimination of each type of sensation. This is done in the parietal lobe. Examples of these sensations are the stereo gnosis, two-point discrimination, and graphesthesia. These senses should also to be evaluated after the extroceptive senses, such as touch sensations and temperature sensing and pain perception, is found to be normal (Griffiths, Barker, Bleiker, Chalmers, & Creamer, 2016).

During the sensory examination, areas that are hyper-sensitive or hypo-sensitive should be marked on the skin; the stimulus used to get this response should also be noted. When any abnormality is noted, the patient should be examined in detail to learn the exact cause of that abnormality and how it will affect the use of heat therapy (Griffiths, Barker, Bleiker, Chalmers, & Creamer, 2016).

 To summarize, heat therapy is highly beneficial to soft tissue injuries and musculoskeletal problems, including osteoarthritis, rheumatic arthritis, and spondylosis, not only because of its physiological effects but its ability to aid in pain management. Another common benefit is its antispasmodic effect, which rapidly reduces muscle spasm, causing relaxation in sub-acute or chronic cases. Thus it is used in muscular spasms like trapezoid spasms, long-term immobilization, arthritis, post-exercise muscle soreness and spasm, and sub-acute muscular strains. Simple forms of heat therapy are highly effective, safe and easy to apply. Heat therapy also has a role in treating many neurological conditions, and in post-surgical cases it may be of use in later stages of rehabilitation. The treatment causes an increase in the blood flow, which aids in tissue repair and because of the increase in oxygen and clearing of metabolites. Heat therapy also has an effect on the extensibility of the connective tissue, which helps increase joint mobility and muscle flexibility (Bigley, 1990).

- **Heat Therapy and Pain**

The gate control theory explains the mechanism of pain – or pain gate - better than any other theory. The small C and A fibers receive noxious stimuli, and at the same time, the large (Aβ) fibers receive less intense mechanical stimuli. The noxious stimuli are carried to the substantia gelatinosa by the C and A fibers, and the pain sensation is felt, which in turn activates inhibition (Guyton, 2008).

Pain comes as nociceptive pain, inflammatory pain and the inflammatory and neuropathic pain of peripheral nerve injury. Extreme heat and extreme cold are noxious stimuli, and a stimulus over an extended period of time may become deleterious (Guyton, 2008).

The exact mechanism of the pain from heating methods is not yet fully understood. This is because the pain can come from many different stimuli or with the same heating stimulus but with a change in the intensity of the heat, and is different in different individuals (Guyton, 2008).

There are two main pain pathways. The first is the peripheral nervous system, with its nociceptors. When stimulated by a thermal stimulus the sensation is carried through the axons of the temperature sensory nerves to the posterior column, along to the thalamus and then the cerebral cortex. The pain pathway includes transduction, in which the nociceptive stimuli stimulate the nociceptors and produce an action potential. The second pain patheway is transmission, in which these stimuli are transmitted as action potentials stimulating the inter-neurons. The perception senses the stimulus in the cerebral cortex and then modulation occurs, in which the inhibitory or facilitator inputs make a change in this nociception (Nicol, 2005).

Thus nociceptors, the pain receptors related to nociceptor pain, are the first unit in the series of neurons related to nociceptive pain. These receptors convert thermal energy to action potentials traveling from the receptors, ultimately to the cerebral cortex, which produces neurotransmitters (Nicol, 2005).

Thus if a noxious heat stimulus is applied, causing an increase in the voltage of the membranes beyond a point of the threshold it causes de-polarisation and ultimately results in the formation of action potential (Nicol, 2005).

CHAPTER 3

The Pathophysiology of Skin

Bhargav Dave, PT, DPT

Learning Objectives:

1. Heat Stress and its effects,
2. Burns and its treatment,
3. Mechanism of heat transfer from heating agent to tissue,
4. Tissue conductivity.

As discussed in the previous chapter, heat is an important component of physical therapy; it aids in rehabilitation after injury and is highly effective in the treatment of musculoskeletal problems. That said, the body's thermoregulatory mechanism is challenged where excess heat is created, and an excessive rise in temperature can lead to serious medical conditions. In other words, if heating modalities are not applied correctly they can lead to complications such as burns, heat rash, and heat stress. Thus, it is critical for therapists to understand how the skin reacts to heat so that burn injury can be avoided (Zhu & Lu, 2010).

It is important to remember the various types of heat transfer, which, as mentioned earlier, work in conjunction with the body's thermoregulatory system. The first kind of heat transfer is radiation, in which the exchange of heat is not from direct contact with the body. Next, comes convection, where the heat is exchanged with the air just over the skin. Last is conduction of heat, using direct contact with an object hotter or colder than the surface of the skin (Mun et al., 2012).

There are several complications that can result from excess or prolonged heat. One of them is heat rash, which develops when blocked or clogged sweat ducts trap perspiration under the skin instead of allowing evaporation. This may ultimately cause blisters, which may be superficial or deep. It may also cause red lumps. The person may feel very itchy, or the condition may remain unnoticed by him/her or even a healthcare professional. Heat rash most commonly occurs in the folds of the skin or wherever there is friction from clothes (Mun et al., 2012).

A deep skin - or miliaria rubra - rash causes red bumps and itching in the affected area. If not tended to, a skin rash may become infected and lead to increased redness, pain and swelling. The bumps may contain pus, and the patient may even suffer from fever and chills. In cases of infection one should also check for any swelling in the adjacent lymph nodes. In a hot and humid climate, heat rash treatment has to be very careful. Also, treatment immediately after intense physical exercise or activity that causes sweat should be considered carefully. For prevention of a skin rash, prolonged overheating should be avoided, as should any ointments or creams that can block the pores. Wearing loose-fitting clothes can be helpful in preventing an excess concentration of heat (Mun et al., 2012).

Heat Stress is a type of heat disorder that occurs when the body loses heat, through conduction, convection or radiation, from the cutaneous blood vessels. When there is a rise in body temperature, either because of a workout or an increase in the surrounding temperature, the cutaneous blood vessels dilate and the pulse rate increases, creating an extra burden on the heart and circulatory system (Parsons, 2009).

When there is excess heat, the body tends to dissipate heat through the skin. It does this by increasing the blood supply to the skin and perspiration. Sudden change in position such as standing, bending down or squatting down can cause dizziness or even blackouts, which can led to other injuries. While we usually think of this occurring while outdoors on a hot day, it is also applicable in physical therapy clinics. The physical therapist should check the patient's condition carefully for dizziness or other symptoms of excess or prolonged heating, and advise the patient against making sudden changes of position after having a heat treatment (Parsons, 2009).

As mentioned earlier, sweating is sometimes the only way of relieving the excess heat. The more area of skin is in direct contact with air, the faster the cooling process; however, it is also important to remember that sweating can cause an individual to lose valuable minerals and bodily fluids. It also causes a decrease in blood volume, which can stress the cardiovascular system. Another potential issue is dehydration, which reduces the amount of perspiration and can cause detrimental effects on the different systems of the body, as well as intravascular coagulopathy (Parsons, 2009).

- **Causes, Symptoms and Treatment of Burns**

Burns are the most common complication associated with heat therapy. The type and severity of the burn depends on the number of layers of skin affected by the heat. Such burns are usually not very severe, and most are preventable if appropriate measures are taken. Burns come in increasing degrees of severity, known as first, second, and third-degree (Aruga & Miyake, 2012).

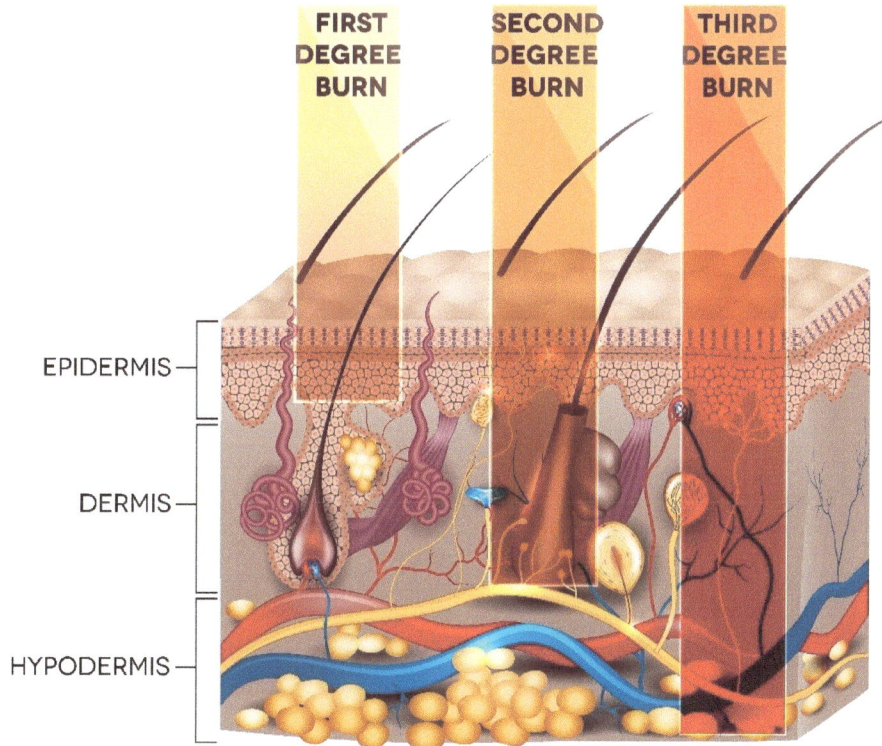

Diagram 2: Degree of Burn

A first-degree burn causes pain and redness on the surface of the skin. One example of this type of burn is sunburn. It can also occur after exposure to infrared or UV radiation during a heat treatment. This type of burn can be treated at home; however, consulting a doctor is necessary if the burn covers a large area or affects the skin over a joint or the face. The best treatment is the application of cold running water immediately after the injury, followed by the application of cold creams or anesthetic to the burn. If necessary, an analgesic and antibiotic can also be administered. The use of ice is not recommended since it can damage the body part. Cotton is also not advisable, as it may stick to the injury and cause an infection (Aruga & Miyake, 2012).

Second-degree burns are more severe than first-degree burns and usually take three to four weeks to heal, depending upon the number of blisters and the area infected. The skin swells and becomes sore and red; it also blisters, which results in peeling (Mun et al., 2012).

Like first-degree burns, second-degree burns are also treated immediately, first by holding it under running water and then applying an ointment or antibiotic ointment to the wound. There is also a small chance a surgery and skin graft may be needed. In any case, a doctor must be consulted when treating second-degree burns, for a proper dressing to protect the burnt tissue from infection and the external environment. Sulfadiazine and/or other antibiotic creams should be applied every time the dressing is changed - usually twice a day. If the burn is large or in a critical area such as the face, groin, buttocks, hands, or feet, it may considered a medical emergency and require more care. As the wound of the burn heals, a fibrinous exudate is formed over the skin. There is usually no scarring, but there is a change in the color of the skin which diminishes over time (Aruga & Miyake, 2012).

Third-degree burns are the most severe form of burn. They cause damage to all the layers of skin, as well as the deeper tissues, such as muscles and tendons, nerves and blood vessels. Such nerve damage burn is associated with the loss of pain sensitivity, and when the affected area is an extremity the blood supply to that extremity is reduced. The symptoms of third-degree burn include charring of the skin, which turns it white in color and leathery in texture. A third-degree burn has a poor prognosis and is associated with many problems, such as infections; shock due to blood loss, and in some case, even death (Aruga & Miyake, 2012).

Other complications arising from these burns are tetanus, hypothermia (caused by excessive heat loss after an injury), and hypovolemia (which occurs due to blood loss during an injury). Tetanus affects muscle contractions as a result of damage to the nerves supplying them (Mun et al., 2012).

Scars resulting from burn injuries are permanent. Scar tissue formation is not preventable; it occurs in the phase of remodeling, which is a proliferative phase of wound healing, therefore, the size of the scar is commensurate with that of the burn. In full thickness burns (those that destroy both the epidermis and dermis), even grafts can lead to hypertrophic scarring. Scars, which are itchy and often painful, can cause suffering on a daily basis, sometimes long after the burn has healed (Aruga & Miyake, 2012).

There are a number of ways in which to deal with the discomfort of scar tissue, including pressure garments. The role of the physical therapist is also important, even in the later stages of rehabilitation after a burn injury. Physical therapy can reduce pain from the scarring and contraction of tissues. The most common sites of post-burn contracture are the hands, upper limbs, and neck, and can have a poor functional outcome. To prevent this, the site should be kept immobilized in a non-contracture position; for example, a cock-up splint can be used to maintain the hand in a particular position and a cervical brace can be used for the neck. There are so many types of braces available in the market for prevention of contracture post burn, one of the gruesome complication of burn. Discussion of which is beyong the scope of this book (Aruga & Miyake, 2012).

In addition to the function implications, scars can also affect the patient emotionally; especially they occur on the face or other visible areas of the body. That said, the importance of appropriate physical therapy treatment, including the prevention of burn injury during these treatment, cannot be overstated. All medical practitioners and therapists must have detailed knowledge of the types of heat through which the different modalities work, the transfer of heat through human body tissues, and their contraindications (Aruga & Miyake, 2012).

- **Burns from Other Sources**

As previously stated, burns can range from very minor to very severe, depending upon the type of burn, the area affected and the depth to which the burn goes. However, burns can also be classified depending upon the source of the injury. Burns can be heat-generated or cold burns, and they can be sustained from electric shocks, chemicals, radiant heat and friction. During treatment with different heating modalities, heat burns -or thermal burns -can result from various sources, such as direct contact with the source of such as hydro-collator packs and hot water bags. Deep-heating modalities such as shortwave diathermy, microwave diathermy, long wave diathermy, and ultrasonic therapy all come in direct contact with the skin and therefore carry a risk of burning if not applied carefully (Aruga & Miyake, 2012).

Electric burns are caused by modalities such as electric heating pads. In all the modalities mentioned above, electric shocks can also result in burns. Chemical burns occur when strong chemicals come in contact with the skin; and radiation burns can result if the radiating heating modality is too close to the area being treated. These modalities can also result in an inhalation burn, in which the latent heat in the form of steam (Aruga & Miyake, 2012).

First-degree, second-degree and third-degree burns may also be classified as superficial partial-thickness burns; deep partial-thickness burns; and full-thickness burns. A superficial partial burn causes damage to the superficial layers of the epidermis, while deep partial-thickness burns injure the dermis of the skin (Mun et al., 2012). Full-thickness burns affect all the layers of the skin and muscles, ligaments, nerves, blood vessels, and – in the most severe cases- the bones. Of all burns resulting from therapeutic modalities, most are caused by hot packs and the most common site is the lower extremities. Hot packs are the most commonly used equipment in physical therapy since they are the cheapest and easiest of all therapeutic modalities; however as they also present the highest risk of burns they must be used with great care ((Aruga & Miyake, 2012).

- **Heat Transfer from Heating Agent to Skin**

With any burn, the severity of the injury depends upon how much heat is passed from the heating source to the skin. How fast the heat is transferred depends on the temperature, the capacity of the source and the length of time it is in contact with the skin surface, the coefficient and temperature of the agent, and the conductivity of the tissues being heated. The capacity of the source to contain heat depends upon the specific heat and the heat capacity of the source of heat. Specific heat is the heat that is required to increase the temperature by one degree of a unit mass substance. Heat capacity is the amount of heat a substance that is the source of heat contains when applied to the skin, which in turn depends upon the heat stored in that material and its temperature at that moment. Thus, the capacity of the source determines how severe the burn injury is. The thermal property of skin is directly related to the functions of the skin. Thus, the conductivity of heat and the thickness of the skin are important for the functions of the skin; the heating rate, pain threshold, formation of blisters. The temperature threshold and the pain threshold depend on the thickness of the epidermis. This is determined through measurements being taken of the thermal pain threshold, surface temperature, time of exposure and the application on a skin surface, which gives the conductivity of the skin. The epidermal thickness is thus determined (Jewo & Fadeyibi, 2015).

- **Temperature**

The initial temperature of the material at the instant of contact is also an important determinant of burn severity. Water heated to 100 degrees cannot be further heated unless it changes its form and becomes vapor. This additional heat, when transferred, can cause burns, as in the case of hot pool baths. The highest degree of the temperature of water alone can cause severe burns. The human body can sustain a temperature of around 46 degrees for approximately six hours; after that body tissues can be destroyed as a result of this excess heat. Contact between a liquid and the skin depends upon the way it is applied (Jewo & Fadeyibi, 2015).

- **Tissue Conductivity**

How tissues conduct heat is also a factor in the severity of a burn injury. The transfer of heat is dependent upon the conduction of heat from the source of that heat through the skin, the body part through which heat is transferred, and the gradient between the skin and the source of heat. Heat conductivity is also dependent upon the creams or oils that are applied to the body, the oils secreted by the body and the water content of the body. A change in blood flow locally causes a vast difference in the transfer and distribution of heat. If the heat transfer is away from the application of heat, this can result in varying degrees of tissue injury (Nielson, Duethman, Howard, Moncure, & Wood, 2016).

Due to its anatomic structure skin is a relatively poor conductor of heat and therefore has a certain resistance to burn injury. The thickness of the skin's outer layer, the epidermis, is consistent all over the body, with the exception of the soles and palms. The epidermis is even thicker in these areas, making them even less likely to sustain a burn injury.

Another factor affecting burn injuries is the depth of the epidermal appendages (i.e. mammary glands, sweat glands, hair follicles and apocrine glands). These appendages differ in individuals depending on their age. Pediatric and geriatric populations have thinner appendages and therefore are more susceptible to full thickness burns. Young adults have relatively thicker appendages, making them less vulnerable to such injury. A burn wound is first assessed for a full thickness burn, which is categorized by three layers of injury: coagulation, stasis, and hyperemia. Coagulation occurs in the area closest to the heat source. It has dead cells because of coagulation necrosis, and the blood flow is absent. This is what causes the surface or the skin to look white (Nielson, Duethman, Howard, Moncure, & Wood, 2016).

Next, is the zone of stasis, which is red in color and may blanch with pressure, which indicates intact circulation, but this flow stops after 24 hours. Petechial hemorrhages are also observed. After two to three days, the intermediate area of stasis also turns white because its dermis no longer has a supply of blood (Nielson, Duethman, Howard, Moncure, & Wood, 2016).

The area of hyperemia is red and blanches on pressure. The circulation is still intact and thus it has a red color. This happens because healing gradually occurs as time progresses to the seventh or eighth day.

After this, there is a transformation that converts the state of stasis to coagulation, which again depends on factors such as progressive dermal ischemia. Chemical mediators such as prostaglandins, histamine, and bradykinin are responsible for this vascular occlusion and cause dermal ischemia to occur. This converts the zone of stasis to a full-thickness burn injury. Different types of prostaglandin have been found in burn wounds, indicating a difference in the vasoconstriction and vasodilatation of prostanoids causing tissue loss in the layer of stasis. In acute or recent burn injuries, there is an increase in oxygen free radicals. For example, xanthine oxidase is the free radical that causes burn edema, which can be treated with xanthine oxidase inhibitors. When 30% or more of the body is burned, chemical mediators such as cytokines are released into the systemic circulation, causing inflammation. There is an increase in the blood flow and an abundance of fluids at the site of burns, which is a systemic inflammatory response. This causes hypovolemia from fluid loss, which results from the lack of perfusion and oxygen supply (Nielson, Duethman, Howard, Moncure, & Wood, 2016).

In third degree burns, hemolysis occurs, which creates a need for blood transfusion to replace blood loss. This also causes a decrease in pulmonary function, without any history of inhalation. In the burnt skin, there is a loss of water due to evaporation causing a heat loss, which can cause hypothermia. Different types of treatment strategy are used to reduce the effects of the thermal injury (Nielson, Duethman, Howard, Moncure, & Wood, 2016).

Non-pharmacologic treatment includes the excision and closing of the wound of the burn, and the treatment of sepsis. Electrotherapeutic modalities used for the treatment of musculoskeletal problems have to be carefully applied, taking into consideration the anatomy and heat transfer mechanism of the skin to avoid complications such as burns and scalds (Nielson, Duethman, Howard, Moncure, & Wood, 2016).

CHAPTER 4

Types of Heat

Bhargav Dave, PT, DPT

Learning Objectives:

1. Different types of heat,
2. Heat transfer and its effect on circulation,
3. Modes of delivery,
4. Coagulative necrosis of skin and its treatment.

As stated in the previous chapter, superficial heating modalities such as hot packs (or hydro-collator packs) are the modality most commonly used modality by physical therapists to treat pain, muscle spasms and joint stiffness, among other things. These hot packs are made of silicate gel packed in a cotton bag. The packs are kept in water in a container that heats it to 71.1 to 79.4°C. This silicate gel has a high capacity for heat absorption. The packs are applied for 20-30 minutes, with layers of towels used as needed. As layers are added, heat flows to the tissue at a lower rate and the temperature rises slowly. Heat conduction increases if there is a leakage of water into the towel.

These treatments, while highly effective, also pose a relatively high risk of burn injury. The risks of other heating modalities include burns from faulty equipments.

Deep heating modalities pose their own risks, including burns from faulty equipment, improper techniques (i.e. the incorrect placement of electrodes), prolonged heating to the patient (or their application to patients with impaired sensations) (Nielson, Duethman, Howard, Moncure, & Wood, 2016) and electric shock. These modalities have electrical energy or currents converted into heat; for example, shortwave diathermy, in which electromagnetic waves are converted to heat, and microwave diathermy and ultrasound, in which ultrasonic waves are converted to heat. This happens when the conversion rate from the current to heat is faster than the heat can dissipate; for example, a short circuit.

This current, if excessive, damages the tissues of the body and can ultimately result in cardiac arrest. Excess current is defined by the type of current, the duration of its application and the voltage associated with it.

A thermal hazard is caused by the passage of excess electrical current. It is a type of short circuit that is caused by faulty equipment. Another hazard comes from using too high a current, which causes the wires to overheat and can result in severe burn injuries. A person can also suffer from electric shock (and possibly burn injuries) while taking any treatment in which the source is applied to the skin. To prevent such accidents, therapists must regularly service their equipment and take care of any issues (Nielson, Duethman, Howard, Moncure, & Wood, 2016).

- **Effect of Heat on Circulation**

Heat increases the blood flow through the body's heat and pain receptors. When heat is applied, the first response is an increase in circulation, which helps to protect the injured tissue and even aid the repair mechanism. The receptors then sense this heat and the person experiences pain.

Modalities such as shortwave diathermy and microwave diathermy work on the principle of electromagnetic waves, which are transformed into heat. They are created when the electrons oscillate due to a temperature increase. Radiant light with shorter wavelengths, such as ultra-violet radiation, cannot be detected by the naked eye. Too much exposure to such radiation can cause sunburn. Radiant light with a greater wavelength than normal visible light, is infrared radiation. Infrared radiation with a wavelength near visible light effects deeper penetration into the tissues, whereas infrared radiation with a deeper wavelength, further from normal light causes superficial heating. Heat forms with greater wavelengths are called diathermies, and these can be converted to heat energy via a conversion heating of the tissues. These forms of energy with longer wavelengths are the shortwave diathermies and the microwave diathermies. Their energy is transferred to heat when they pass in the body and for their transfer, no medium is required (Houghton PE, 2010).

- **Heat Transfer**

When superficial heat is used, the transfer of heat stops at the surface of the skin because the layer of fats (adipose tissue) insulates the deep tissues. Transfer of heat to those tissues depends on three types of heat transfer: conduction, convection and conversion heating.

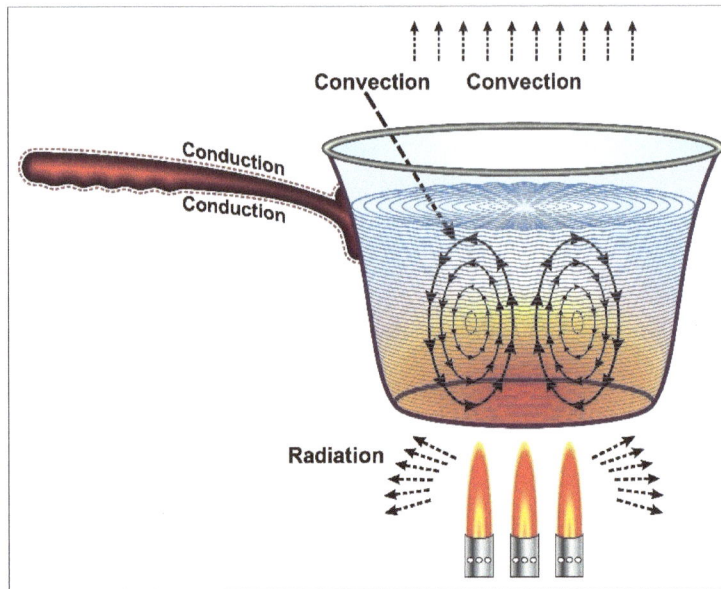

Diagram 3: Types of Heat Transfer

Conductive heating is where the transfer of heat is the result of direct contact. Such heating does not cause any change in the medium that conducts heat; for example, the superficial heat that results from placing such things as hot packs, hot water bags, and electric heating pads directly on the skin.

Convection heating causes movement in the medium (i.e. air or fluid) that transfers the heat. Examples of such heat transfer are whirlpool baths, paraffin wax baths, and hydrotherapy.

Conversion heating is where another form of energy, such as light or sound, is converted into heat; for example, a heat lamp that converts light energy into heat on the surface of the skin.

Heat transfer also depends upon several other factors, such as the surface area to be treated, the temperature of the skin at the time of treatment and the rate at which these temperatures increase (Chapman, Liebert, Lininger, & Groth, 2007).

Indications for Using Different Types of Heat for Therapeutic Purposes

Conductive history is widely used by physical therapists, often in form of hot packs. As mentioned earlier, hot packs are widely used in treating muscular spasm, joint pain and stiffness and muscle pain, backaches, cervical and lumbar spondylosis, delayed-onset of muscle soreness, frozen shoulder, and many sub-acute or chronic cases of soft tissue injury such as sprains and muscle strains. They are also beneficial for abdominal muscle cramping such as cramps during menstruation. That said, there are a contraindications associated with each type of heating; for example, paraffin wax baths, which is a type of conductive heating modality, cannot be used to treat open wounds (Chapman, Liebert, Lininger, & Groth, 2007).

Convective heating includes fluidotherapy and hydrotherapy. Fluidotherapy is highly beneficial in cases of pain from arthritic conditions in small joints (i.e. rheumatoid arthritis); chronic post-fracture joint stiffness prior to mobilization; and stiffness in the shoulder/hand syndrome. It also provides a sedative effect and pain relief to patients on an exercise regime for pain and stiffness in the joints from conditions such as sickle cell anemia. Hydrotherapy (whirlpool) can be used in the treatment of infected wounds (i.e. irrigation) (Chapman, Liebert, Lininger, & Groth, 2007).

Another therapy is the contrast bath, which creates hyperemia for therapeutic purposes in the treatment of rheumatoid arthritis or pain related to the sympathetic system. There are contraindications associated with this type of heating as well; for example, it should not be used in the presence of open wounds, as these wounds are not supposed to get wet. There are also other special precautions that need to be taken, such as continuous monitoring of patients with psychiatric illness. Hubbard tanks increase the body temperature, which can be an issue in patients with hypersensitivity to heat. This type of therapy should also not be used on pregnant women(Chapman, Liebert, Lininger, & Groth, 2007).

Conversion heating which includes treatment modalities such as infrared lamps, plays a role in treating musculoskeletal conditions such as muscle spasms and many orthopedic conditions, as well as cases where direct contact with a heat source is contraindicated (i.e. skin discontinuity and rheumatoid arthritis). Any radiant heat is contraindicated when there is acute inflammation, hypersensitivity to radiant heat, or in patients with decreased sensations and bleeding disorders (Chapman, Liebert, Lininger, & Groth, 2007).

Conductive heating is used extensively in physical therapy clinics and is also being taught to patients for use at home. That said, if not administered properly this type of heating can also lead to complications, such as burns, drying of the skin, and –depending on the weight of the modality - hampering local blood supply to the treated area. This also is possible through uneven distribution of pressure on the uneven anatomical surface being treated (Cetin, Aytar, Atalay, & Akman, 2008).

- **ThermoTherapy**

This category, which includes both superficial and deep heating modalities. Superficial heating modalities cause an increase in temperature and blood flow to the area, as well as the supply of oxygen and nutrients; they also accelerate the proliferation of fibro blast cells and endothelial cells, all of which hasten the healing process. ThermoTherapy also increases the elasticity of connective tissue and relaxes the muscles by reducing the spindle and gamma efferent firing rate, which relieves spasms. The contraindications for these modalities are thrombophlebitis, or deep vein thrombosis, acute inflammation, impaired circulation of the part, impaired sensation of the part, infections such as tuberculosis (local), malignancies, hemorrhages, and skin diseases (Cetin, Aytar, Atalay, & Akman, 2008).

Heating from modalities with electromagnetic waves, as in short-wave diathermy, microwave diathermy, and laser therapy, is therefore used for many medical ailments. Many developments have occurred recently because of their effectiveness in treating many musculoskeletal conditions. Therefore, knowledge of heat transfer mechanisms and the mechanics of heat in the skin is of utmost importance. The study of Biothermomechanics includes heat transfer, burns, and physiology. The mechanical response to heat and the pain levels related to it and effectiveness of each heating modality must be understood.

The difference between the complications of the effects of temperature on burns and thermal stress caused because of treatment with various modalities has been presented here. Thus we see that the thermo-mechanics of the skin are very complicated. The effect of blood perfusion causes a significant difference in temperature distribution, producing a thermal stress. Microwave diathermy and laser treatment cause thermal stress only in the superficial layer, the epidermis, and not in the deeper layers (Cetin, Aytar, Atalay, & Akman, 2008).

Precautions

It is critical for physical therapists to be aware of the risks of superficial heating modalities and safeguard against them. Such modalities should not be used on pregnant women or patients with cardiac issues, for example; they should also not be used on the carotid sinus or in conjunction with topical irritants. Metal items such as jewelry, keys and belts must be removed before treatment; and metal implants must be avoided. Possible complications of superficial heating include burns, dizziness, bleeding of open wounds, and skin discontinuity (J. Petrofsky et al., 2013). The prevention of such complications is possible by taking few precautions, such as testing the skin sensitivity of the patient (i.e. for heat and cold) prior to treatment. While using hot packs, the heating pad should be covered with a thick layer of toweling to avoid burns (keep in mind that any water leakage from hot packs increases the temperature of the towel in which it is wrapped and should be checked intermittently during treatment). The patient should also be checked for any signs such as redness, blisters, excess sweating, or any sign of burns. The risk of burns is greater with this type of heating because the heat is concentrated superficially, as the subcutaneous fat below the skin acts as an insulator. Lying on hot packs produces excess pressure that may compress the pack, causing water to ooze out and cause burns. This is very painful to the patient, due to the latent heat in hot water being transferred to the body (J. Petrofsky et al., 2013).

- **Paraffin Wax Bath**

Another type of conductive heating is the paraffin wax bath, which is useful in treating the stiff joints of rheumatoid arthritis, burns, systemic sclerosis, and the finger and hand stiffness of the shoulder/hand syndrome. Paraffin wax is applied to the smaller joints of the hands and feet. This paraffin is melted in a wax bath container which is controlled thermostatically. Two methods are used for wax application: the dip method, in which the hand or foot is kept in the paraffin bath and removed when a thin layer has formed over the skin. This is repeated until a thick layer is formed over the skin. The second is the immersion method, in which the part to be treated is immersed in the paraffin bath for 20-30 minutes. This method transfers heat from solid or liquid paraffin. The transfer of heat is reduced in this method, because of the solid paraffin glove formed during the initial immersion. This type of conduction heating produces a significant rise in the superficial skin temperature, but a decrease in the temperature of the subcutaneous tissue (Cetin, Aytar, Atalay, & Akman, 2008).

- **Fluidotherapy, Hydrotherapy and Whirlpool**

Fluidotherapy and hydrotherapy are examples of the convection type of heating. In this method, temperature-controlled air is passed through a solid such as glass beads. The part that is to be treated, such as the hand or foot, is immersed. This is a type of superficial dry heating, and the temperature is the same as the hot air that is passed in. In hydrotherapy, there is the complete immersion of the part in a hot tub, whereas whirlpool baths are more useful for partial immersions. Hydrotherapy is excellent for treating draining wounds. In such a case, the container in which the part is immersed is sterilized. Another more type of convection modality is the moist air cabinet. Moist air containing water vapor at a certain temperature is blown over the patient, giving superficial heating beneficial for the entire body, heating the skin and superficial tissue. It is helpful in treating back-muscle spasms, and in arthritic conditions involving many joints throughout the body (Chapman, Liebert, Lininger, & Groth, 2007).

- **Conversion Heating, or Radiant Heat Therapy**

In conversion heating, high-energy photons penetrate the tissues. One example is radiant heat, which is effective for treating many skin conditions, including psoriasis (J. Petrofsky et al., 2013). When the heat is applied, these high-energy photons travel through the tissues and are converted into heat. This transferred heat is superficial because of its longer wavelength. Another type of these lamps is the ultraviolet, infrared lamp using a Carborundum heating element. To achieve maximum benefit the source of the heat is placed between 50 and 65 centimeters from the patient, for at least 20-30 minutes, although this will depend upon the particular patient's sensitivity. Infrared radiation is also utilized for reflex vasodilatation if excess vasospasm has occurred due to pain. Radiant heat is effective for the treatment of many skin conditions, including psoriasis (Chapman, Liebert, Lininger, & Groth, 2007).

- **Deep Heating (Conversion Heat)**

This is a form of energy which, when converted into heat inside the body, produces deep heating within the tissues as well as on the surface of the skin. At the surface, the rise in temperature is at the cellular level, through direct and reflex action. There is an increase in the blood flow through dilation of the blood vessels or capillaries, and they are quite permeable, so there is a change in metabolism. All this can lead to a change in the pain threshold and decrease in muscle spasm and muscle relaxation, due to vasodilatation. This can be used in chronic conditions and can accommodate large joints. When acute inflammatory processes are occurring, deep heating requires extreme care, because it can obscure inflammation. In mild heating, a temperature rise also occurs in tissue away from the site of application. When the temperature rises slowly, reflex vasodilatation occurs. Modalities such as short-wave diathermy, ultrasound, and microwave diathermy work on these principles of deep heating. All of these modalities cause a rise in temperature in the tissues through relative heating (or the amount of energy being converted to heat at any given location). The practitioner can select a modality that gives the highest temperature at the affected area without increasing it beyond the tolerance level of the patient. This rise in temperature is dependent on the type of heat, its conductivity, and the length of time (Chapman, Liebert, Lininger, & Groth, 2007).

Modalities such as short-wave diathermy can heat superficial muscle through a certain frequency of an induction coil, and can be used in heating the pelvic organs too, with an internal electrode. It also may be utilized for pelvic muscle spasm. Similarly, microwave therapy applied at a certain frequency can thoroughly heat the muscle. Ultrasonography is specifically used for heating parts surrounded by thick, soft tissues such as ligaments, muscle tendons, tendon sheaths, fibrous scars, and nerve tissue. On the other hand, microwave or shortwave diathermy radiation can provide effective heating to deep subcutaneous tissue, and help in the relaxation of superficial muscles. Microwaves can also be utilized for selective heating of muscle. . Shortwave diathermy can be selectively used over the pelvic organs, for coccygeal muscle spasm and in conditions such as of chronic pelvic inflammatory disease (Chapman, Liebert, Lininger, & Groth, 2007).

- **Dry Heat and Moist Heat**

There are several differences between moist heat and dry heat; for example, moist heat is more effective in treating pain. Also, while both dry and moist heats are both used to treat post-exercise soreness, they have different methods of delivering relief. With most chemical heat wraps, for example, the transfer of heat is fast and can be applied for more than two hours. With dry chemical heat wraps, the heat transfer is very slow. In addition, moist heat, when applied immediately after exercise, preserves muscle strength, reduces pain and prevents alteration in the elasticity of the tissues. Preservation of muscle strength after exercise is an increase in blood supply to the tissues. This increases the metabolism and speeds removal of waste products. The increase in tissue metabolism is doubled, with an increase of temperature by two degrees, which helps in tissue healing. Hence, if the application of the heat after exercise is for a long period, the blood flow remains constant for a long time, which helps in tissue healing and recovery from damage due to exercise, such as in delayed-onset muscle soreness (Brock Symons et al., 2004).

They also differ in their capacity to penetrate the tissues. The research shows that moist heat penetrates well and further into the tissues than dry heat because the transfer of heat through moist heating travels faster through the skin. It is the same with moist and dry air. When the air is humid, the transfer of heat is much more rapidly than with dry air conditions. So penetration is deeper and can be used for deep injuries (J. Petrofsky et al., 2013).

- **Short-wave Diathermy (SWD)**

Shortwave Diathermy is a deep heating modality that uses high radio frequency currents in order to produce heat. Essentially, it creates an electromagnetic field that relieves pain and hyperemia, as well as the reduction of muscle spasms (which occurs because of an increase in blood supply). To treat a larger area, a transverse technique for application of SWD is adopted. The concentration of heat is at the mid-point of applied electrodes. Tuning of this modality is required for the appropriate application. The temperature should be such that the patient feels a soothing heat, and he or she should be monitored throughout. The treatment should be administered on a wooden chair or table and usually lasts for 20 minutes. There are two further methods of application of SWD. They are the "condenser method" and the "inductive coil method" (Chapman et al., 2007).

- **Microwave Diathermy**

This deep heating modality also works on the principle of electromagnetic radiation. It selectively heats the parts with a higher concentration of water. It has some the same benefits as SWD, (i.e. pain relief) and uses similar wavelengths; however, the frequencies used in microwave diathermy are greater than those used in shortwave diathermy. The lower frequency gives the effect of selective heating of the muscle, and less heat is transferred to subcutaneous fat. This mechanism is of greater advantage in cases where selective heating is required. Like SWD, microwave diathermy can cause complications such as burns, which occur as a result of perspiration brought on by the selective heating technique. Treatment with microwaves is also applied for 20 to 30 minutes (Chapman et al., 2007).

- **Ultrasound**

Ultrasound is yet another deep heating modality that works on the principle of high-frequency vibrations, albeit those at a range inaudible to humans. The frequency of the ultrasound used for therapy is usually between 0.8 and 3 M Hz and are produced by a piezo-electric effect. This energy is applied to the crystal, which vibrates at this high frequency and generates waves which when passed through the tissues are converted into heat. They can also give a non-thermal effect if required. The treatment uses pulsed or continuous waves, depending upon how long the patient has had the injury, and lasts between five and 10 minutes; however, adjustments to the intensity and duration can be made depending upon the condition. The patient should feel comfortable when the heat is generated. Ultrasonic therapy produces pain-relieving effects, increases blood flow to the area and cell permeability and relieves muscle spasms. It works through the conduction of the peripheral nerves. A complication involved with this type of deep heating is the production of a hot spot, which may be caused if the ultrasonic head is not moved continuously on the area of application (Chapman et al., 2007).

- **Heat Administration and Burns**

As mentioned earlier, these treatments, while rather simple and easy to administer, carry risks. To avoid these risks, the first step is collecting a detailed history and clinical evaluation prior to treatment. This includes an investigation of any underlying pathology that could be a contraindication to heat therapy. The patient should be evaluated for dysesthesia, any site of malignancy, an open wound or inflammation, diabetic neuropathy or any other neurological condition, and sensory deficits (hypo-sensitivity to heat). The patient's mental state should also be evaluated (Jewo & Fadeyibi, 2015).

When home treatment is required, it should be monitored by a medical practitioner so that the patient does not fall asleep during the treatment and/or the heat is not applied for too long.

When excess heat is applied, there is an increase in blood flow due to the dilatation of the capillaries. The permeability of these capillaries also increases, and plasma leaks from the capillaries. Since the plasma is released into the surrounding interstitial tissues, there is a reduction in plasma concentration, which can result in hypovolemic shock. The more significant the burn injury, the greater the loss of plasma (could be fatal if not addressed in timely manner), and may require a blood transfusion (Jewo & Fadeyibi, 2015).

Infection is the most common complication of burn injury. Such infections do not occur at the time of the injury, since the same heat that caused the burns also cleanses the area of any microorganisms. Without proper post-injury care, however, these wounds can be affected by bacteria and can even lead to life-threatening conditions (Jewo & Fadeyibi, 2015).

While managing burns, special attention must be paid to any blisters that have formed by the plasma that lies between the burnt epidermis and the dermis. This plasma contains proteins and therefore it serves as a medium for bacteria to grow and multiply. An improperly treated wound can also be infected by viruses and fungi that can lead to sepsis. Other systemic infections such as pneumonia are also common and are caused by organisms such as staphylococcus aureus and pseudomonas. The most common fungus that affects burn wounds is Candida Albicans. This threat is even greater when the body is immune-suppressed. Suppression of the immune system can be specific or nonspecific. When the immunoglobulin is affected, sepsis occurs after approximately one week (Jewo & Fadeyibi, 2015).

Burn wounds are primarily treated with bactericidal creams and in the case of systemic infection, oral or intravenous antibiotics. Dressings must also be changed regularly in order to keep the wound sterile and prevent the growth of organisms. However, in burns, they cannot be used this way since they are of no use at the site of sub eschar (Jewo & Fadeyibi, 2015).

Massive burn injuries take a long time to heal, and the catabolic phase is extended. In injuries other than burns, catabolism is shorter and wounds are covered faster. Nutrition also plays an important role in recovery. The body rebuilds through a lot of wear and tear mechanisms, and calorie and protein requirements are very high (Jewo & Fadeyibi, 2015).

CHAPTER 5

The Effectiveness of Various Types of Heat in the Treatment of Pain

Bhargav Dave, PT, DPT

Learning Objectives:

1. Literature review,
2. Deep tissue heating vs. superficial tissue heating,
3. Moist heat vs. dry heat,
4. Use of heat in sterilization,
5. Effectiveness of MWD & Therapeutic ultrasound.

Physical therapeutic modalities are used to create ideal environment for injury repair by preventing the inflammatory process and breaking the pain cycle. As such, the decision to use a particular modality highly depends on the location, type and severity of the injury, as it relates to contraindications (Escoffre & Bouakaz, 2015). For example, thermotherapy can be contraindicated for tendinitis during the initial – or acute - phases of therapy. It is also critical to monitor the individual's progress throughout to be certain that the appropriate modality is being used.

The previous chapter touched on the frequencies used by various deep heating modalities. Within that category there are several distinct therapeutic tools –sound, light, thermal and mechanical – that physical therapists can use to treat a broad array of conditions. These physical agents play an integral role in the reduction of pain and joint swelling; they also restore one's mobility and increase the blood flow to the wounded tissues. For instance, thermal modality uses ultrasound to treat various musculoskeletal conditions like the tendonitis and muscle strains.

According to Boucaud (2004), this therapeutic procedure benefits a patient by reduction of local inflammation and stimulates tissue healing by increment of blood supply in relatively superficial tissues. The phonophoresis type of therapy uses ultrasound to drive in topical medications through the skin to treat localized inflammations. Electrotherapeutics is used to reduce pain and inflammation, thereby promoting tissue healing, stimulates nerve or muscle function, and sensory integrative therapy (Carmen, et al., 2004). Therefore, physical therapy substantially assists in managing the recovery of soft tissue injuries and disorders, enhances a patient's functional range of motion, muscular strength, improvement of body posture and mechanics; it also restores balance.

In relation to deep tissue heating techniques, deep heat is emitted when energy is converted into heat as it navigates through body tissues. As Draper (2010) puts it, the energy sources used include the use of high–frequency currents-shortwave diathermy, electromagnetic radiation such as microwaves, and use of ultrasound by means of high-frequency sound. Therefore, the temperature distribution in the tissues heated by any of the mentioned mechanisms results from a pattern of relative heating which is equal to the amount of energy to heat at any prescribed area. A practitioner is highly advised to select a heating modality that produces the highest temperature at the site of concern without any form of exceeding (Michlovitz, Bellew, & Jr, 2011). Given this, the main goal of this form of treatment should be accepted by the patient having provided them with adequate and/or complete data to be at a position of making an informed decision.

- **Deep tissue heating verses superficial tissue heating**

Superficial tissue heating is used to warm up muscles and is often applied in form of hot packs, paraffin, infrared radiation, or fluid therapy. The effectiveness of superficial tissue heating is experienced especially when the technique is applied simultaneously with a low-load static stretch that improves the flexibility of shoulder and muscle as compared to deep tissue heating (Fatemi, 2009). On the other hand, the application of deep-tissue, ultrasound techniques substantially helps in healing connective tissues.

Superficial tissue heating is also very effective when used as a relaxing and palliative modality for patients suffering from tension or hyper-myotonicity. Furthermore, it can be used for treatment of increased extensibility of collagen, decreased joint stiffness, and relief of muscle spasm. When using paraffin bath treatment, there should be no open wounds, acute episodes of inflammatory arthritis or rashes in the treatment area. Apparently, this type of superficial tissue heating is effective in treating distal extremities and chronic injuries-to the wrists, hands and feet (Mo, Coussios, Seymour, & Carlisle, 2012). Therefore, for affectivity and efficiency purposes hydro-collator pack, type of superficial heat, should be used as an adjunct to enable an active exercise program. Fitzgerald, Malik, & Ahmed (2011) state that this type of treatment suits acute phase therapies where the goal is to reduce pain and inflammation. Similarly, deep heat modalities are used a variety of pain conditions and reduction of muscle spasm by use of transcutaneous electrical nerve stimulation (TENS) and electrical stimulation effectively. Basically, the modalities are effectively used in the treatment of chronic pain conditions and reduce pain by fifty percent.

In contrast to deep tissue heating modalities, the increased cutaneous blood circulation from superficial heating significantly causes a cooling reaction because it eliminates the heat that is applied externally (Suri, 2008). Conversion heating involves the conversion of an energy form such as sound into another like heat (Harris, 2005). In this case it allows for the production of superficial heat by means of heat lamps and radiant light bakers with heat being moved when the conveying medium is converted to heat energy at the skin. For instance, therapeutic cold also known as cryotherapy has a primary influence of cooling tissue.

Overall, both deep tissue heating and superficial tissue heating modalities use the thermo factor in facilitating therapy process. Research by Zhou (2015) has proved that the usage of these modalities is effective in facilitating healing process if they are used properly and accurately. However, it is important to note that early application of heat can exacerbate tissue damage in an acute injury and significantly prolong the healing process. Noticeably, the key aspect in which the practitioner should take into account while performing physical therapy is to understand how and when to use heat (Suri, 2008). This helps the clinician to use care and safe measures during treatment.

Use and effectiveness of moist verses dry heat

Both the moist and dry heat therapies are types of superficial heat therapy. Moist heat therapy, which is often used for the treatment of pain, stiffness and secondary muscle spasm in chronic arthritis and muscle spasm on posterior neck (Nadler, Weingand, & Kruse, 2004), seems to be more effective than dry heat in providing deeper penetration of body tissue at the same temperatures. Moist heat also alters tissue temperatures more rapidly and obtains a more dynamic reaction from temperature receptors (Giombini, et al., 2007). Many patients who undergo moist heat therapies report greater relief from pain. It speeds up recovery by increasing blood flow to the targeted area, thus causing increase in blood flow that brings about fresh blood and takes away the toxins that may slow down the healing process.

To ensure the therapy program delivers help rather than harm, practitioners should avoid using heat on a fresh injury because it may increase the pain and swelling of the wound; heat therapy should not be used on patients who have circulatory problems or are unconscious, so as to prevent burning or damaging the skin. Dry heat therapy draws moisture out of the skin by use of electric. Most people find it convenient to use dry heat technique; however, it could potentially disadvantage a patient because it can dehydrate the skin. Therefore, obviously the technique is not suitable for people who have dry skin problem.

Use of Heat in Sterilization

There are significant differences between dry heat and moist heat therapies with regard to sterilization of materials. According to Block (2001), moist heat sterilization works with high water pressure through the use of an autoclave instrument. Compared to dry heat sterilization, the temperature of this technique is lower but with high pressure it assists with effective moist heat sterilization. This effectively facilitates elimination of structural proteins and organism's enzymes which consequently die (Starkey, 2013). Particularly, moist heat technique is significantly used for heat sensitive substances through which heat is permeable.

On the other hand, dry heat sterilization uses heated air or fire. This method uses higher temperatures as compared to moist heat and is therefore more effective for killing organisms. This destructive oxidation method assists in destroying large contaminating bio-molecules like proteins. In this case it requires the temperatures to be maintained almost an hour to kill the most resistant spores. It effectively works best on substances such as syringes, metal instruments and glassware (Hawkes, Draper, Johnson, Diede, & Rigby, 2013).

Effectiveness of Microwave diathermy and Therapeutic ultrasound

Diathermy is a therapeutic treatment prescribed for joint conditions such as rheumatoid arthritis, musculoskeletal, and osteoarthritis (Alves, Angrisani, & Santiago, 2009). The process delivers a high-frequency electric current through shortwave, microwave or ultrasound to produce deep heat in body tissue. The heat is tremendously used to increase blood flow and relieve pain; it is used to seal off blood vessels and destroying of abnormal cells (Shakoor, Rahman, & Moyeenuzzaman, 2008). In application, microwave diathermy does not apply direct to the body but rather the current from machine allows for the body to produce heat from within the targeted tissue. This way, it promotes blood circulation that significantly improves flexibility in stiff joints and connective tissue. Thus, due to reduction of pain the patients suffering from arthritis are more capable of increasing their range of motion (Kaltenborn, 2002). Microwave diathermy uses microwaves to produce heat in the body; further it is used to evenly warm deep tissues without burning the skin. However, the therapy technique does not penetrate deep muscles it is thus suitable for locations that are closer to the skin like the shoulders.

Ultrasound diathermy employs high-frequency acoustic vibrations in which when stimulated through the tissue, they are converted into heat. This type of therapy is importantly useful in the delivery of heat to selected musculatures structures because it conducts differing sensitivity of various fibers to the acoustic vibrations; in that some of them are more absorptive and others are reflective (Robertson & Baker, 2001). For instance, in subcutaneous fat, little energy is converted into heat however in the muscle tissues there is higher rate of conversion to heat. As such, the therapeutic ultrasound device produces a high-frequency alternating current which is converted to into acoustic vibrations. When conducting treatment, the device should be moved slowly across the surface being treated. Generally, ultrasound is an effective agent in therapy process because of its unique application of heat (Foley, Little, & Vaezy, 2008). However, it should be used only by the practitioner who is completely aware of its potential risks and the contradictions for its application.

Hyperthermia is often induced by microwave diathermy in the management of muscle and tendon injuries. Hyperthermia significantly raises the temperature of deep tissues using electro-magnetic power. As such, microwave diathermy is used in the control of superficial tumors in presence of convectional radiation-therapy and chemotherapy. Therefore hyperthermia induced by microwave diathermy into body tissue can potentially stimulate repair process, increment of drug activity allow for efficient relief from pain and removal of toxic wastes. Moreover, it enhances local tissue drainage, induces permeability in the cell membrane and increases metabolic rate. Noticeably, microwave diathermy cannot be applied in high dosage on edematous tissue over wet dressing or close to metallic implants in the body due to the fact that it may result to local burns. Similarly, the use of hyperthermia is only safe if the temperatures are kept under 45 degrees Celsius, otherwise it does not a sufficient way to predict the damage that it may cause.

In summary, all the discussed physical therapy techniques are efficient in treating different types of injuries or body discomforts. However, research emphasizes on keen observation on comprehending how they are supposed to be used because if otherwise they could result to adverse damage to body tissues. Additionally, it is important to note that these advances incorporate use of heat or electricity to facilitate their effectiveness thus is essential for the practitioner to regularly monitor the patient and ensure that in every step of the process he/she consults with the patient about their condition. Lastly, due to the amount of risks or hazards that can accrue due to the usage of physical therapy techniques it is required that the patient should understand fully and consent to the type of physical therapy that is applied. Having highlighted the key concerns discovered in the research conducted it would be safe to state deep tissue heating and superficial heating modalities, moist heat and dry heat therapies, and microwave diathermy and therapeutically ultrasound are effective and play an integral role in delivering treatment depending on the medical prescribed suitability.

CHAPTER 6

Therapeutic Modalities

Bhargav Dave, PT, DPT

Learning Objectives:

1. Literature review,
2. Diathermy vs. Ultrasound,
3. Modalities,
4. Deep heating vs. superficial heating,
5. Use of different heat and stretching,
6. Heat and exercises,
7. Use of heat and wound care.

Rehabilitation in physical therapy aims at a return to activity and functional independence after an injury. This includes first the relief of pain, spasms and stiffness and increasing the range of motion. The next phase of rehabilitation is aimed at recovery of muscle strength, endurance and power. The use of modalities for this recovery phase is a good adjunct to exercise. In the acute and sub-acute stages of injuries, they help reduce pain and muscle spasm and promote early tissue repair and healing, to take the patient quickly to the stage of functional independence, by treating the root cause of pain.

The use of modalities is indicated where the modality is going to be beneficial, and contraindications for modalities are conditions in which the modality may worsen the situation. Indication and contraindication can be present for the same condition; heat can be indicated in a later stage of recovery but contraindicated in the early stage of inflammation. So the application of a modality and its selection depends upon evaluation of the condition and a detailed history related to the ailment (Chapman, Liebert, Lininger, & Groth, 2007).

Thermotherapy has developed into many different modalities, such as deep and superficial heating modalities beneficial to all the musculoskeletal conditions, with their different physiological effects. Some modalities have a greater advantage of easy accessibility, low cost, many can be used at home if well monitored, and they can bring long-term benefits. Their effect on tissue healing is unique and the patient feels very comfortable and relaxed, apart from the therapeutic effects it administers. The patient can get back to their routine pain free, and can avoid too long a break from work (Chapman, Liebert, Lininger, & Groth, 2007).

Heat therapy can give unique effects compared with pharmacological drugs, which will only help in reducing the swelling and in relaxation of the muscles and pain reduction Heating modalities help in the early restoration of function, working in synchrony with the different phases of healing and does not cause further tissue damage by the early loading of the tissue with drugs (Chapman, Liebert, Lininger, & Groth, 2007).

It is best to treat first the symptoms of soft tissue injury, such as muscle spasm, pain and joint restriction. These modalities are very effective in muscle spasms that protect the part, such as spasms of the back muscles in back strains. Once the patient is out of the spasm, strengthening the back muscles can begin, depending upon the orthopedic condition. The modality is selected according to the area of muscle spasm. For example, on a small area of muscle spasm, hot packs or even a deep-heat modality such as shortwave diathermy can be administered. But if the area to be targeted is larger, such as post-exercise muscle soreness or the entire back, full immersion in a hydrotherapy or whirlpool bath can be effective (Chapman, Liebert, Lininger, & Groth, 2007).

The effectiveness of heat therapy on a joint's range of motion is another great advantage of this therapy. When the joint is stiff from trauma post-fracture or due to some form of arthritis, deep heating modalities such as ultrasound or shortwave diathermy can be of great advantage because their deep penetration into the tissues. The swelling around the joint subsides and the spasm surrounding it is lessened, reducing the stiffness. Ultrasound also increases the elasticity of the connective tissue and relieves stiffness. Hot packs can also be very helpful prior to stretching, increasing the flexibility of the joint. The joint injuries that can be treated with these modalities include all types of arthritis, post-fracture stiffness, degenerative conditions, tennis elbow and golfer's elbow (Chapman, Liebert, Lininger, & Groth, 2007).

The heating modalities described in this book can be used either alone or in conjunction with other techniques and exercises to reduce pain, accelerate the healing process, increase muscle flexibility and relieve muscle spasms through relaxation. The most commonly used modality is the hot pack because of its easy availability and easy application with great results. Moxibustion is also an important heating tool, the only disadvantage being the risk of burns due to incorrect application (Rand, Goerlich, Marchand, & Jablecki, 2007).

Early and appropriate intervention is critical for any musculoskeletal condition, as it can speed the return to normal activity levels and help prevent recurrence. After diagnosing the ailment (including the nature of the injury and the stage of healing), the physical therapist will prescribe the appropriate therapeutic heat modality (including the intensity), the frequency of the energy used, the duration of each treatment, and rehabilitation exercises in the office and at home. The treatment program is then modified as needed throughout, according to the stages of rehabilitation. Phase one is the "reducing the pain" stage, meaning increasing one's range of motion, building isometric strength, reducing muscle spasms, and decreasing any inflammation. The next stage of rehabilitation is the "return to activity" phase. Heat modalities are usually beneficial in this phase, especially when used with other forms of treatment such as rehabilitation exercises (Giombini et al., 2007).

Through the process, the precautions to be taken should be noted and followed meticulously (Brucker, Knight, Rubley, & Draper, 2005). Indications, contraindications, use, and precautions are of prime importance for a physical therapy plan of care. This has to be communicated to physicians, nurses and other health care practitioners.

Various heating modalities have gained importance as rehabilitation equipment. Short-wave diathermy is the most well-known modality in physical rehabilitation. Diathermy works on the principle of high-frequency currents converted to electromagnetic waves, causing deep heating. Heating modalities include microwave, shortwave and long wave diathermy, and differ in radio frequency. The penetration depends upon the wavelength. Long wave diathermy has the deepest penetration of all types of diathermy, because of its longer wavelength, but is almost redundant because of its higher risk of burns. Short wave diathermy is the most widely used and is very safe with good tissue penetration. Diathermies can stimulate collagen for repair, and can therefore effectively promote tissue healing and can enhance the healing of bone and cartilage. Therefore, it is very effective in treatment of all types of arthritis, such as rheumatoid arthritis and osteoarthritis. Shortwave diathermy consists of both pulsed and continuous types of diathermy and can be used for deeper tissue penetration and produces a quick rise in temperature. The penetration is exactly the same as ultrasound. So when the desired result is to increase the tissue temperature with deeper penetration to cover a larger area, the role of pulsed short-wave diathermy is important. It can be used to improve the extensibility of the soft tissues along with stretching. It is also helpful for increasing long-term flexibility (Rabini et al., 2012).

- **Continuous and pulsed diathermy vs ultrasound**

Both pulsed and continuous short-wave diathermy provide heating effects dissimilar to ultrasound. When compared to ultrasound, diathermy has some unique advantages over ultrasound. The waves of shortwave diathermy are not reflected as with ultrasound, where the bones and tissues reflect the waves. There is, therefore, less risk of burns causing hot spots. Ultrasound is considered to be safer than diathermy, but this is a misconception, since every modality has its own advantages and disadvantages, safety measures and risks of complications. Ultrasound engages the therapist during treatment, whereas short-wave diathermy once started can be simply monitored. When these modalities are used over a long period, therapists can observe specific tissue healing (Rabini et al., 2012).

Shortwave continuous diathermy produces more heat from more energy, so can be more effective, with its higher heating. But because it produces more heat energy, there is a high chance of a significant rise in temperature in a short time, which can soon become uncomfortable and risk burning (Rabini et al., 2012).

- **Shortwave Diathermy**

Shortwave diathermy is a deep-heating modality in which heat is produced by the conversion of electromagnetic waves into heat as they pass into the tissues. Its advantage is that it can treat a large area in one session. Electromagnetic waves are produced at a frequency of 27.12 hz, produced by high radio-frequency electrical currents. Shortwave diathermy offers the physiologic effects of pain relief, hyperemia and a sedative effect. There is an increase in blood flow, causing relaxation of muscle spasm (Yildiriim, Ucar, & Ones, 2015).

  o **Application**

There are various application techniques depending upon the area to be treated for maximum advantage. One is the transverse technique, which covers a large treatment area between the two electrodes where the heat is concentrated before tuning is done. The patient's circuit is tuned to resonate in such a way that the frequency of their circuit is same as the frequency of the machine. For maximum therapeutic advantage, the temperature of the tissue should be taken to 40 degrees and the duration of the treatment should be 20 to 30 minutes. Treatment should be performed on a wooden table (Yildiriim, Ucar, & Ones, 2015).

The other method is the called the condenser. In this application, the heat is concentrated between the two electrodes covering the area to be treated. These two electrodes act as the capacitors. If the patient moves, the amplitude of the concentrated heat can be affected, so the patient has to be monitored. Felt or plastic spacers are used in this method (Yildiriim, Ucar, & Ones, 2015).

The next method of application is the induction method, in which the inductive coil heats the superficial muscles and also joints with a thin layer covering the joint. In both the condenser and inductive methods, a towel should be kept nearby to wipe off any perspiration to avoid local concentration of the heat, and the patient should be still and should not move. The machine output is adjusted so movement of the patient does not change the impedance of the circuit or increase current flow. In either case it can cause burns. It is very important that the machine is tuned at low power according to the patient's heat tolerance, and that the readings are noted (Yildiriim, Ucar, & Ones, 2015).

  o **Indications**

Indication for shortwave diathermy includes musculoskeletal pathology. It produces the physiological effects of deep heating on the tissues. The deep heating modality selected depends upon the desired effect. Shortwave diathermy is effective on musculoskeletal pain, inflammation, and muscle spasms, sub acute and chronic cases of sprains and muscle strains, and soft tissue conditions such as tendinitis, tenosynovitis, and bursitis. It is highly effective in adhesive capsulitis because of the deep heating it causes. The appropriate use of diathermy is dependent upon the position of electrodes around the treatment site. It also depends upon which part is to be treated and the type of tissue involved. Where impedance from the tissue is high, the heat produced by the machine must increase.

o **Contraindications**

Contraindications for shortwave diathermy include malignancies, in which the deep heating may increase metastasis, and tuberculosis, in which the condition worsens if there is increase in the infection. It is also contraindicated where there are metallic implants or cardiac pacemakers in the body that may interfere in the circuit. Pregnant women are at risk because of the deep heating effects, and it is also contraindicated in patients suffering from arteriosclerosis, thromboanginitis and phlebitis(Lammertink et al., 2015).

o **Precautions**

Special precaution must be taken where women have metal implants such as a intra-uterine device, or during menstruation. Also patients wearing metal ornaments or carrying metals such as coins, keys or belt buckles should remove them before the therapy, as metals may interfere with the circuits and cause shocks. Patients wearing contact lenses should remove them before the therapy. Special care must be taken while treating geriatric patients or small children (Lammertink et al., 2015).

o **Complications**

Short-wave diathermy may cause the common complication of all heat modalities, burns. These may occur through application of improper techniques, not monitoring the patient intermittently during sessions and use of equipment that is not well maintained (Lammertink et al., 2015).

- **Microwave Diathermy**

Microwave diathermy is also a type of electromagnetic radiation modality and has the special advantage of heating the deep tissues with higher water content only, so causing selective heating of the tissues. Its physiologic effects are similar to that of shortwave diathermy: hyperemia, relief of pain and muscle spasm and a sedative effect due to increased blood supply, causing an increase in local metabolism. The frequencies at which microwave works are 915 MHz, and 2456 MHz. The wavelength of the microwave diathermy is the same as shortwave, but the frequency is much higher so it is easier to focus. A lower frequency is still selected for the treatment of selected muscles, and less heat is transferred to subcutaneous tissues (Wong, Schumann, Townsend, & Phelps, 2007).

o **Indications**

Owing to these physiological effects and selective heating, microwave diathermy can be effectively applied to muscle contractures to improve the flexibility of the collagen fibers of the muscles. Thus, it can be applied prior to stretching the muscles in contracture. Secondary muscle spasm is another condition in which microwave diathermy can be put to use. Such spasm is generally present over the trigger points. It is also used on the smaller and superficial joints with a thin layer of skin, such as in hands and feet (Wong, Schumann, Townsend, & Phelps, 2007).

○ **Application**

The equipment has a director that focuses the microwaves over the area to be treated. It can allow viewing of the site of treatment. The distance of the director can be altered at the treatment site to reduce or increase the amount of heat. So the equipment should be placed where the patient gets the appropriate heat level at which they are comfortable. The duration of the treatment is generally 20 to 30 minutes (Wong, Schumann, Townsend, & Phelps, 2007) .

○ **Complications**

As with short-wave diathermy and microwave diathermy, there is a burn risk if the proper technique is not applied, and a burn risk from localized perspiration in microwave diathermy because of its selective heating method (Wong, Schumann, Townsend, & Phelps, 2007).

○ **Contraindications and precautions**

Contraindications are the same as that in shortwave diathermy. Additional precautions must be taken while using microwave diathermy for synovitis, and infections, whether they are local or systemic. Special precautions must be taken over bony prominences (Wong, Schumann, Townsend, & Phelps, 2007).

- **Ultrasonography**

Ultrasound utilizes high-frequency sonic waves or sound waves, mainly for tissue healing, which takes place at a cellular level. The superficial tissue covering the targeted part turns warm when it is applied for 5 to 10 minutes.

○ **Indications**

Primarily used in soft tissue injuries such as ligament sprains, muscle strains, tendonitis, joint stiffness and also as temporary pain relief, since it assists early healing and tissue repair, bone fracture healing, tendon injuries, venous and pressure ulcers, and surgical incisions.

Ultrasound is used in osteoarthritis of the knee, because of its known effect on the extensibility of the connective tissue, and so can be used for treating contractures in osteoarthritis and thus prevent deformity. The usefulness of ultrasound is due to its physiological effects. Ultrasound consists of ultrasonic waves which, when they enter the body, are converted into heat, which is generally concentrated in a smaller localized area. A larger area can be targeted by other deep heating modalities such as shortwave diathermy. Thus the injuries exclusively treated with ultrasound are: strains and sprains with a small pinpoint area that can be targeted with the deep penetration effect of ultrasound, rotator cuff injuries, ligament sprains in ankle and knee and strains in rhomboids or other scapular muscles, and quadriceps or hamstring strains (Anderson, 2012).

○ **Contraindications**

These include malignancies and tumors, joint replacement surgery because of the metal inside, pacemakers, implants of eyes and breasts, and some areas such as reproductive organs (Anderson, 2012).

○ **Special precautions for the prevention of complications**

The ultrasound has to be kept rotating continuously to avoid potential burns to the part treated. An appropriate amount of medium for the waves to penetrate has to be ensured, or this coupling medium may increase heat to the skin, causing burns (Anderson, 2012).

○ **Application**

The parameters of the machine such as intensity, frequency and duration give special effects in particular conditions. Ultrasound gives both a thermal and non-thermal effect, using pulsed and continuous modes.

Continuous ultrasound gives a heating effect on the tissues, whereas pulsed ultrasound applied at an acute stage of soft tissue injury stimulates the process of healing, and works on a cellular level by making a difference to membrane permeability. It uses two frequencies, a higher frequency and lower frequency. Higher frequencies can be beneficial for superficial tissues such as the patellar tendon (Anderson, 2012).

Ultrasound with a lower frequency is helpful for the deep penetration required in cases of muscle spasm and muscle and ligament sprains. More research is needed in order to determine the effectiveness of this therapy in treating orthopedic conditions is needed.

• **Phonophorosis**

This is another treatment using the ultrasound machine, using high-frequency ultrasonic waves for the passage of medicine through the tissues. The medicines used for this treatment are usually topical analgesics or steroids. These can be used in painful conditions, where anesthetics or steroid injections are otherwise used. An NSAID is mixed with the medium and ultrasound is applied, at an intensity of one or two watts, to aid penetration (Masiero, 2008).

• **Sonochemotherapy**

Ultrasonic waves are used for the administration of certain drugs through the tissues. The drug can be administered locally with the help of microbubbles produced by the ultrasound, producing physiological effects. They increase the permeability of the cells, or plasma membrane, and also vascular permeability, to transfer the drug. The same mechanism is also used for administration of chemotherapy drugs,or sonochemotherapy (Masiero, 2008). Ultrasound increases soft-tissue extensibility and may be an effective adjunct in the treatment of knee contractures secondary to connective tissue shortening (Hawkes, Draper, Johnson, Diede, & Rigby, 2013).

- **Deep heating vs. superficial heating**

Superficial heating modalities heat only the skin and subcutaneous tissue, not the subcutaneous layer of fats that a deep heating modality reaches. The subcutaneous layer acts as an insulating material against the transfer of heat. In superficial heating, there is an increase in cutaneous blood-flow to the part. Heat transfer occurs in three different forms as mentioned earlier; conduction, convection and conversion. In conduction heating, the heat transfer occurs from one point to another, with no movement or change in the conductive medium, and direct contact is made with the source of heat (Hawkes, Draper, Johnson, Diede, & Rigby, 2013).

Examples of such heating are hydro-collator or hot packs, electric heating, and paraffin wax baths. In convection heating, the transfer of heat occurs with a significant change in the medium of heat transfer from hydrotherapy, whirlpool baths, and fluidotherapy (Hawkes, Draper, Johnson, Diede, & Rigby, 2013).

Radiant heat is conversion heating, in which one form of energy is converted into another form; heat. Modalities with this type of heating include infrared lamps and UV lamps, where light or radiations are transferred into heat, which is focused on the skin. The physiologic effects from this type of heating depend upon the initial temperature of the tissues, the rate at which this temperature increases the size of the area to be treated, and treatment duration for the rise of temperature (Hawkes, Draper, Johnson, Diede, & Rigby, 2013).

- **Hot Packs**

Hot packs, or hydrocollator packs, are a type of superficial heating modality that works on conductive heating for its transfer of heat. They consist of silicate gel in a cotton cover, and are kept in thermostatically controlled water containers. The silicate gel absorbs heat from the water. Its capacity to absorb heat is very high.

- o **Application**

They are applied wrapped in a towel forming 6 to 8 layers and placed over the skin of the part to be treated for 20 to 30 minutes. Heat is transferred through conduction to the superficial tissues.

Wrapping a towel over the pack controls excess transfer of heat. However, if there is leakage from the hot pack, the temperature of the towel increases, causing increased transfer of heat. To avoid such leakage, check the temperature every five minutes and avoid having the patient lie on hot packs, which may force water out and cause burns (Hawkes, Draper, Johnson, Diede, & Rigby, 2013).

Hot packs are useful for many conditions: pain, muscle spasm, pain in abdomen during menstruation, superficial thrombophebitis, and muscle stiffness and tightness.

○ **Advantages**

The most important advantage of using a hot pack is its easy and effective use. Its application is simple with easy availability. It can be used as a home therapy if well monitored. There are different forms of hot pack. They include Kenny packs, rubber water bottles, and electric heating pads, which also produce moist heat that gives efficient heat transfer (Hawkes, Draper, Johnson, Diede, & Rigby, 2013).

Electric heating pads can be a danger because of the risk of shock if not covered with an insulating material. Risk may also occur if the patient falls asleep, because heat produces an analgesic effect, but ultimately may result in burns. Care is also to be taken in patients with altered sensations or patients with mental challenges (Hawkes, Draper, Johnson, Diede, & Rigby, 2013).

• **Paraffin Wax bath**

Paraffin wax baths are a modality in which the transfer of heat occurs through conduction. It is used in some specific cases such as hand stiffness, which may be post fracture or from shoulder/arm syndrome. It effectively avoids contracture from long-term pain and stiffness. It is generally used for areas such as hands and feet or smaller joints. It contains paraffin wax mixed with liquid paraffin and heated in a wax bath container to a specific temperature, which is usually the melting point of the paraffin (Hawkes, Draper, Johnson, Diede, & Rigby, 2013).

○ **Application**

The area to be treated is washed with soap and water. There are two methods of application; the dip method and the immersion method.

Dip method

In this method, the hand or foot to be treated is held in the paraffin wax to form a thin layer and then removed from the wax bath when it has adhered to the skin. This procedure is repeated until a thick layer of wax has formed, like a glove. The heat is preserved if the patient's hand is covered with the towel for 15 to 20 minutes. The paraffin is then removed and replaced in its container. This type of superficial heating retains heat for some time in the small joints, which become more mobile and stiffness reduces. After the part is dipped and covered with plastic or a towel, a range of motion exercises are performed (Hawkes, Draper, Johnson, Diede, & Rigby, 2013).

Immersion method

Here the part to be treated is immersed in wax for 30 minutes. Heat is transferred from the solid as well as liquid paraffin in the container. Since the solid paraffin forms a thick layer over the immersed part, the heat transferred through the liquid paraffin is lower and forms more slowly, to act as an insulator and protect the part from excessive heat (Khan, 2013).

This method increases the skin temperature significantly, and significantly decreases the temperature of the subcutaneous tissue. The advantage of this method is that if water were used at the same temperature, the heat transferred would very high (Khan, 2013).

o **Indications**

Mobility can be restored in a stiff hand from shoulder/hand syndrome with the application of paraffin wax for 30 minutes, because the heat is long lasting. It is also useful for the chronic stiff joints of rheumatoid arthritis, post-burn cases with stiff joints and cases of scleroderma (Khan, 2013).

o **Complications and special precautions**

Deep vein thrombosis and haemorrhagic conditions can worsen with this type of heating. It can be risky in those with impaired sensation of the skin. Acute inflammatory conditions are not to be considered for this form of therapy. Direct contact with broken skin should be avoided. Its application over the reproductive areas is also contraindicated (Khan, 2013).

• **Fluidotherapy**

This superficial heating modality is a type of convection heating. It consists of solid glass beads into which thermostatically controlled warm air is blown, and this produces a semi-solid heating environment. This creates a dry heat. The temperature of the dry heat is the same as that of the blown dry air. The part to be treated, such as hand or foot, is immersed and heated superficially (Khan, 2013).

o **Indications**

Fluidotherapy is utilized for pain relief; it is used for arthritic small joints, and prior to mobilization in stiff joints, sickle cell anemia, and for relaxation post exercise.

A similar therapy is hydrotherapy, which uses total immersion in a big tub of hot water. Hydrotherapy has the advantage that it can be also used where there are draining, infected wounds, if proper precautions are taken to sterilize the tub.

Very similar to fluidotherapy and hydrotherapy is whirlpool therapy, which is generally used for partial immersion of the extremities.

- o **Indications, contraindications and special precautions for convective therapy**

In hydrotherapy, where there is total immersion of the body, care has to be taken that there is no rise of temperature above 40 degrees. In partial immersion, heat should not exceed 46 degrees Celsius. Total body immersion has a relaxing effect, as it lowers the blood pressure because of peripheral blood pooling. These therapies are not applicable where open wounds are present. Application of these therapies is not possible for conditions involving temperature sensitivity, such as multiple sclerosis, SLE, renal failure and pregnancy.

- **Moist air cabinet**

Another convection modality is the moist air cabinet. The patient sits in the cabinet, through which moist air is passed, thereby causing superficial heating over the whole body.

- o **Indications**

This modality is excellent for large area, for example when the entire back muscles go in spasm. It is also very helpful in polyarthritic conditions.

- o **Precautions**

The increase in temperature has to be checked and monitored every five minutes. If the patient is sweating heavily, the temperature control must be adjusted.

- o **Contraindications**

These are similar to convective heating modalities such as fluid- and hydrotherapy.

- **Contrast baths**

These produce therapeutic hyperemia, which can be of great advantage for sympathetic nerve control, such as for rheumatoid arthritis, sprains or strains causing effusions. In this convective heating method, a difference of 25 degrees Celsius is maintained between hot and cold. The hot water is maintained at approximately 40 to 43 degrees, and cold water at 15 to 20 degrees Celsius. Its effects are achieved by hyperemia, which is achieved by a ratio of 10:1 minutes. The part is immersed in hot water for 10 minutes and then cold water for one minute. This process is repeated for 30 minutes (Page et al., 2014).

- **Whirlpool baths**

This is therapy in which the effect of heating is combined with the effect of massage, given by its turbines. It is especially useful for increasing the range of motion of a stiff joint by making use of the buoyancy of water, which is helpful for the movement performed. If the range of motion is restricted due to injury, swelling that remains in the sub-acute or chronic stage can be immersed in water and 'alphabet' exercises are done. With assistance of the buoyancy of the water, a swollen part can be moved and the joint stiffness reduced. In the whirlpool bath either the extremity that is affected or the whole body can be immersed (Page et al., 2014).

- ○ **Precautions**

When the whole body is treated with this therapy, the temperature of the water must be monitored so it does not to go beyond the desired level of 102 degrees or the comfort level of the patient. The duration of the treatment should not exceed 20 or 30 minutes, since a longer time can cause peripheral pooling of the blood, lowering blood pressure in some patients (Page et al., 2014).

- **Radiant heat modalities**

Here the transfer of heat is through conversion heating. This type of heat is produced when high-energy photons pass through the tissues and this energy is transformed into heat energy. The penetration of the photons is superficial, producing superficial heating, because of the wavelengths of the photons.

There are different types of radiating heat, depending upon the wavelengths of the photons. This spectrum ranges from short wavelength, infrared radiation, to photons with longer wavelengths that produce ultra violet rays. Higher heat is produced by shorter wavelength photons that generate greater penetration of the tissues.

- ○ **Indications**

This type of conversion heating produces greater relaxation muscle spasm. It is also advantageous for conditions in which direct contact with the heating surface is not indicated, such as rheumatic arthritis or when skin breakdown is present, such psoriasis, and when reflex vasodilatation is required if vasospasm occurs.

o   **Application**

The lamp is placed 50 to 60 centimeters from the part to be treated for the radiant heat to be beneficial. The treatment duration is 20 to 30minutes, and the duration is depends upon how long the patient feels comforting warmth. Intensity of the light is dependent upon the type of reflector and the distance of the source of light from the treated part.

Laser therapy is also called "light amplification" because of the emission of radiation. The laser form of heat radiation causes a very specific and controlled emission of light from the source. These lasers emit low light radiation, which is less than the light emitted by the main light source in the room. Laser radiation is a controlled form of emission, and the level of milli watts is much less than the level of light in the room, which is at a level 70 to 100 watts. The laser has a chamber containing a medium for the transfer of rays. This chamber has mirrors on both sides of the chamber, parallel to each other. One of those mirrors is slightly open. This medium is excited by electricity (Jain & Sharma, 2014).

o   **Limitations**

In open wounds, some convective or conductive heating, such as fluidotherapy or paraffin wax baths, cannot be used. Also, surgical wounds cannot be treated with hydrotherapy. Patients with sensitivity to light cannot be treated with radiant heating. Also, radiant heat is not applicable for patients with bleeding disorders, altered sensation sensitivity or inflammatory conditions.

In hydrotherapy, a total dip in water can increase the core temperature of the body. Thus we need to be cautious in cases of renal failure and SLE, since the body becomes more sensitive to the rise in core temperature. This is also true with pregnant women.

- **The Use of Deep Heating and Superficial Heating Modalities Prior to Stretching**

Over recent years, flexibility of the tissues has become an important prerequisite for the avoidance of musculoskeletal injuries. To attain this, physical therapists make use of many heating modalities prior to a program of stretching, to improve joint flexibility. These modalities have a physiological effect of increasing extensibility of the connective tissues, which in turn leads to increase in their flexibility. The use of these heating modalities prior to stretching helps decrease muscle spasms due to injury, by the relaxation of the tissues because of a decrease in activity of the muscle spindles. Their use also increases bloodflow through the dilatation of the capillaries, and there is an increase in the local metabolism of the tissues. Superficial heating in particular improves extensibility of the tissues, reduces pain, restores mobility and decreases the viscosity of the tissues. Deep heating has the advantage of reducing the sensitivity of nerves, which relieves pain.

A study regarding the effects of superficial heat and deep heat has shown they increase the range of motion in joints through an increase in flexibility of the muscles around the joint. They also increase the flexibility in the surrounding tissues. Deep heating is understood to cause more improvement on the extensibility of the tissues than superficial heating or cryotherapy. Ultrasound prior to stretching has made a difference in the treatment of stretching. Athletes also make use of heat therapy in conjunction with their regular stretching routine. The choice between superficial and deep heating modality depends on the patient's condition and preferences. There was an observation which demonstrated a direct relationship between the heat applied before and during stretching sessions and the flexibility of connective tissues.

- **Effects of Deep Heating Modalities on Musculoskeletal Conditions**

  o **Adhesive Capsulitis**

Commonly known as "frozen shoulder," this causes a marked restriction in shoulder movement, associated with pain, causing limited activity and restricting function. Heating modalities play an important role in reducing pain and increasing the flexibility of the tissues around the shoulder. They are most effectively used before mobilization of the shoulder. Other beneficial effects include improved sleep, as they relax spasming muscles and increased joint flexibility. In studies comparing electrotherapy with non-heating modalities, placebo and no treatment, patients reported the greatest results from the electrotherapy, citing relief of pain and increased flexibility, range of motion and function.

A combination of two modalities, such as ultrasound iontophorosis and continuous shortwave diathermy have proved especially effective for treating adhesive capsulitis; so has using one heating modality and a non-heating modality, such as TENS. Manual therapy also works well in conjunction with these therapies. In fact, when compared with hydrocortisone injections, combination therapy proved more useful in improving the range of shoulder motion, therefore functional performance (Dehghan & Farahbod, 2014). Low level laser treatment was very useful in relief of pain and thus improving function. Deep heating was useful for short-term pain relief and improving range of motion (Mayer et al., 2005).

- **Heat therapy for low back pain**

Acute low back pain is the most common form of physical ailment, especially among those with a sedentary lifestyle and office work. A study of the use of heating modalities on these patients showed it helps in relieving muscle spasms, lumbar canal stenosis, chronic PID, spondylysthesis and lumbar spondylosis were treated with heat therapy prior to other forms of treatment.

Low back pain can be acute, sub-acute or chronic and is often treated with a combination of medicines (i.e. analgesics, anti-inflammatory muscle relaxants) and physical therapy modalities. The heating modalities in physical therapy have been proved to be very beneficial in the treatment of low back pain for long-term benefit in superficial tissues, the muscles and the joints deep inside.

Acute low back pain is very important to treat, to avoid restriction in daily activities. About 75 percent of people suffer from this very often. To reduce this incidence or to treat acute low back cases for an early return to activity, it is important to access the most effective treatments, including thermotherapy. Core strengthening for the back muscles brings the most effective long-term benefits in chronic low back pain.

Thus, heating modalities are one of the most effective treatments on low back pain and, along with core strengthening exercises, useful in chronic cases, with the advantage of long-term pain relief. Heat modalities for back pain include short-wave diathermy, hydro-collator packs, hot water bottles, infrared radiant heating, and convective heating or hydrotherapy (total immersion) (Kloth, 1995). Heat therapy and cold therapy are both equally effective in low back pain.

- **Use of therapeutic modalities in wound healing**

There are certain conditions in which only the right environment for healing will help, or the wound condition may deteriorate (McCulloch, 1995).

Some heating modalities and ultraviolet radiation can be useful in enhancing the process of wound healing. Ultraviolet radiation can cause hyperplasia and stimulate epithelial activity, increase granulation tissue formation and removal of dead metabolites, and have a detrimental effect on harmful organisms such as bacteria that may prolong the process of tissue healing. Heating modalities increase the circulation of the affected tissue, increasing the oxygen level in the tissues, thus enhancing wound healing. When these modalities are not used properly there is a high risk of a further damage to the tissues (Houglum, 2016).

Heating has also proven extremely effective on ulcers, including arterial and venous ulcers, non-healings ulcers and those that are slow to heal. In deep heating modalities such as ultrasound, fibroblasts are stimulated and mast cells de-granulated, which helps with inflammation. Hydrotherapy is also uniquely helpful for tissue healing, because the water helps in the removal of debris and help increased blood flow to the ischemic wound, thus promoting healing of the ulcers (Anderson, 2012).

CHAPTER 7

Influence of Age, Race, Gender and Diabetes on the Skin Circulation

Jerrold Petrofsky, Ph D, JD

Learning Objectives:

1. Literature review,
2. Interaction between stimuli on vascular endothelial cells,
3. Gender and endothelial function,
4. The influence of diabetes on skin circulation,
5. Race, lifestyle, and endothelial function,
6. Interaction between Age and Diabetes.

When people are exposed to a thermally neutral environment, skin blood flow averages about 5% of cardiac output. However, during whole body exposure to heat, skin blood flow can increase to about 8 L/m (Rowell 1974). In glabrous (non-hairy) skin (e.g. palms, plantar aspects of the feet and lips) cutaneous arterioles are innervated by only sympathetic adrenergic vasoconstrictor nerves (Fox and Edholm 1963; Johnson 1986; Rowell 1977). Cutaneous blood flow in glabrous skin is mediated by vasoconstrictor tone and the effects of local metabolites and effectors such as skin temperature and pressure (Johnson 1986; Johnson and Brengelmann 1986; Johnson and Proppe 1996; Rowell 1977). In hairy, or nonglabrous skin, found in the majority of the body, 3 separate sympathetic pathways are involved in the control of the skin blood flow. Adrenergic vasoconstrictor nerves reduce (constrict) skin blood flow. Cholinergic and nitrogenic nerves elicit vasodilatation in skin blood vessels through the release of either acetylcholine or nitric oxide respectively (Charkoudian and Johnson 1999b; Johnson and Proppe 1996; Rowell 1977; Jennings and Donald 2008).

As was the case for glabrous skin, local effectors such as metabolites and local skin temperature or pressure can also result in changes in skin blood flow. Thus, the control of circulation in the skin can be divided into generally 2 types of control, the local response to metabolites and other processes such as local pressure or shear stress on the blood vessel wall and neurogenic control through the sympathetic nervous system. Synapses from the sympathetic nervous system release chemical transmitters that elicit a response from vascular endothelial cells, causing vasoconstriction or vasodilatation of the surrounding smooth muscle through chemical transmitters.

Nitric oxide is one of the most potent vasodilators in the skin. It is released by vascular endothelial cells. The bioavailability of nitric oxide is a balance between nitric oxide production and degradation.

Nitric oxide can be degraded by reaction with some oxides and but largely super oxides caused by a variety of pathologies including ageing and diabetes yielding, instead of nitric oxide, triple oxygen bearing molecules such as peroxy nitrate (Rahman et al 2006, Mates 2000). Increased oxidative stress can potentially be moderated via activation of NADPH oxidases or xanthine oxidases in the vascular wall (Hare 2004, Kozak et al 2005). Instability in ENOS can also liberate oxygen instead of nitric oxide (33). Decreased bioavailability of L-Arginine is also correlated with ENOS uncoupling in vivo (Fostermann et al 1994). Thus, increases in oxidative stress such as that seen in diabetes and due to cigarette smoking may not alter nitric oxide production via NOS pathways but the effect is the same by reducing bioavailability. The result is impaired vasodilatation (Rahman et al 2006, Mates 2000). With a reduction in nitric oxide bioavailability, there is a preponderant vasoconstriction in blood vessels as seen in hypertension, cardiovascular disease, and diabetes (Giordano 2005, Griendling and Fitzgerald 2003a, Griendling and Fitzgerald 2003b), raising cardiac work and blood pressure.

Another vasodilator substance released by vascular endothelial cells is a prostaglandin, prostacyclin (PGI2) (Lenasi and Struci 2008). Especially in younger subjects, both nitric oxide and prostacyclin are released as a result of sympathetic vasodilator nerve activity (Lenasi and Struci 2008). However, associated with ageing, prostacyclin release is reduced and nitric oxide becomes the predominant vasodilator (Malty and Petrofsky 2007, Holowatz et al 2003, Haendeler 2006). In younger subjects, in one study, at least 60% of acetylcholine mediated vasodilatation was still preserved after combined ENOS and COX inhibition (Lenasi and Struci 2008). While this shows an important role of nitric oxide and prostacyclin I 2 mechanisms in the regulation of the cutaneous circulation, it points to the other substances that are can also be released by vascular endothelial cells, especially in younger individuals, which can also mediate an increase in blood flow (Lenasi & Struci, 2008).

The effect of local temperature on skin blood flow is mediated by vascular endothelial cells that line the blood vessels. In response to an increase in skin temperature, cutaneous blood vessels dilate by a temperaturedependant mechanism (Kellogg 2006). Maximal skin blood flow is reached at skin temperature of about 42°C for about 30 minutes (Taylor et al 1984). Local vasodilation is a biphasic response with an initial vasodilation followed by a prolonged plateau. The mechanism of local cutaneous vasodilation involves both local neuromechanisms (axon refluxes) as well as local generation of nitric oxide. The two mechanisms are independent of each other (Minson et al 2001). The local sensory component (initial response to local heat) is mediated through local sensory nerves mediated by release of substances such as Substance P (Minson et al 2001; Pergola et al 1993). The sensory arm of this response is vanilloid type 1 receptors on local sensory nerves (Stephens et al 2001). This activates a local axon reflux causing an increase in skin blood flow (Stephens et al 2001).

The prolonged plateau phase to local temperature is mediated by nitric oxide. It is therefore attenuated by the nitric oxide inhibitor LNAME (Kellogg et al 1999; Minson et al 2001). Since activation of the enzyme nitric oxide synthetase involves heat shock proteins, heat shock protein inhibitors (HSP 90) reduce the sustained increase in skin blood flow to local heat (Garcia-Cardena et al 1998).

Shear receptors are also present on the surface of vascular endothelial cells. These shear receptors, through a prostaglandin mediated mechanism; activate the enzyme nitric oxide synthetase. This involves the activations of TRPV-4 voltage gated calcium channels which then, through activation of nitric oxide synthetase cause the production of nitric oxide (Hinds et al 2008). These same TRPV-4 channels are also involved in the prolonged response to muscle temperature as described above. The local increase muscle temperature also increases influx of calcium through TRPV-4 channels which then activates nitric oxide synthetase. Thus, voltage gated TRPV-4 calcium channels are involved in a number of different processes to activate endothelial nitric oxide synthetase.

Obviously, the endothelial cell is also sensitive to other substances that won't be discussed in detail here. However, receptors on the endothelial cells for ATP, histamine, bradykinins, and other prostaglandin compounds also are involved in mediation of vasodilator and vasoconstrictor substances released from the vascular endothelial cells that influence the surrounding smooth muscle.

- **Interaction between stimuli on vascular endothelial cells**

From a global perspective, the interaction between vasodilator and vasoconstrictor inputs into the vascular endothelial cell is obvious. For the sympathetic nerves, if more action potentials occur on vasoconstrictor nerves than vasodilator nerves, the balance will be more release of vasoconstrictor substances such as prostaglandin H2 than vasodilators such as nitric oxide and the predominant tone of the smooth muscle will be vasoconstriction. If, on the other hand, there is a small vasoconstrictor tone from the sympathetic adrenergics and a large flood of acetylcholine from sympathetic vasodilator nerves, then the predominant tone of smooth muscle is relaxation. However, there appears to be more than this simple interaction that takes place with the vascular endothelial cells.

Recent studies (Petrofsky et al 2008a) have shown that when multiple stimuli are applied simultaneously on vascular endothelial cells, the response is not just additive but is nonlinear. For example, electrical stimulation (the use of electric current across the skin) can induce the release of nitric oxide and hence vasodilation (Petrofsky et al 2008a, Petrofsky 2007b). However, if the same current is applied when local skin temperature is cool (<25°C) there is no increase in blood flow in the skin to the electrical. If skin temperature is warmed to 30°C, there is a small increase in blood flow. At a skin temperature of 35°C there is a very large increase in blood flow to this stimulus. Thus, when various effectors are added together, the total response can be synergistic. Even changing skin temperature from 35 to 36°C causes a much larger increase in blood flow then increasing skin temperature from 34 to 35°C. This is seen with a variety of stimuli such as, for example, the interaction between local and global heat.

Heating of the entire body while using ice to locally cool the skin abolishes the skin blood flow response to sympathetic vasodilator nerves. Warming the skin, but keeping the skin dry reduces the blood flow response of the skin in a nonlinear way to local temperature. Many of these differences may be caused by interaction on the TRPV-4 calcium channels on the vascular endothelial cell. Looking at local temperature alone for example, raising skin temperature from 25 to 35°C causes a nonlinear increase in calcium influx into vascular endothelial cells as a function of temperature (Petrofsky et al 2008c; Petrofsky et al 2008f). These receptor channelsthen, if nonlinear in their response, would provide a nonlinear increase in ENOS activation. Thus, in complex situations such as global heating of the body, local heating of the skin and simultaneous hydration or dehydration of the body, the skin response becomes somewhat unpredictable in terms of the blood flow change associated with multiple stressors. This is confounded further by other endothelial agonists and antagonists such as estrogen.

- **Gender and endothelial function**

The menstrual cycle is divided into the follicular and luteal phases. These phases are characterized by fluctuations in the reproductive hormones estrogen and progesterone (Charkoudian and Joyner 2004). The follicular phase can be subdivided into early follicular and late follicular phases and the luteal phase can be subdivided into early and late luteal phases. In the early follicular phase (days 1-7), after the onset of bleeding, estrogen and progesterone concentrations in the blood are low while in the late follicular phase (days 8-14) estrogen levels increase due to the effect of follicular stimulating hormone (FSH) (Charkoudian and Joyner 2004). During the late luteal phase (days 15-21), levels of progesterone and estrogen increase due to the formation of the corpus luteum and in the late luteal phase (days 22-28), both hormones gradually decrease reaching their lowest levels at day 28 of the menstrual cycle (Lloyd et al 2000, Bern et al 2004). The fluctuations in estrogen and progesterone, in turn, influence the thermoregulatory system in premenopausal women (Petrofsky et al 1976, Charkoudian and Johnson 1999c, Charkoudian 2003). Core temperature increases by an average of 0.3 to 0.5°C during the mid-luteal phase altering the threshold for sweating and skin blood flow and the response to exercise or to whole body heating (Petrofsky et al 1976). The fluctuation in female reproductive hormones has direct effects on circulation in the skin (Al Malty, Petrofsky, and Suh 2007). For example, local cooling of the hands of premenopausal women to 15°C induces excessive vasoconstriction during the luteal phase compared to the response in the follicular phase of the menstrual cycle (Cankar, Finderle, and Struci 2000). There was also attenuation of the vascular response during reactive hyperemia of the forearm after arterial occlusion (Petrofsky et al 1976, Bungum et al 1996).

Furthermore, skin sensitivity to sodium lauryl sulfate is altered during the menstrual cycle; skin is more irritable on the first day of the menstrual cycle than during the 9th or 10th day (Agner, Damm, and Skouby 1991). Further, the intensity of existing skin diseases changes throughout the menstrual cycle.

For example, atopic dermatitis exacerbates during the first day of the menstrual cycle (Kemmet 1989). In addition, resting skin blood flow and muscle blood flow is modulated with the menstrual cycle and during exercise (Petrofsky et al 2007a). These effects provide telling evidence that changes in the microvasculature response to local stimuli may be caused by some local vascular mechanisms rather than central mechanisms. Specific receptors for estrogen have been identified throughout the arterial system (Sarrel 1990, Guo et al 2005). These receptors are believed to play a major role in modulating the skin blood flow response to local stimuli based on the plasma estrogen concentration. The fact that many of these changes are lost when women are administered the birth control pill (Petrofsky et al 1976) and in older women (AlMalty et al 2008a) is further evidence of the presence of estrogen receptors in the cardiovascular system. In addition, the modulation in the resting skin blood flow is further altered during exercise (Petrofsky et al 2007a).

Clinical evidence strongly suggests that estrogen plays a role in both changing blood flow and angiogenesis of blood vessels (Anal et al 2007). Endothelial progenitor cells (EPC) isolated from peripheral blood has been shown to incorporate into foci for neovascularization in the adult; this effect varies during the menstrual cycle (Asahara et al 1997, Shi et al 1998). EPC's are generally derived from bone marrow and mobilized in response to tissue damage and/or cytokine stimulation (Heissig et al 2002, Ceradini et al 2004). Mature vascular endothelial cells express at least two different estrogen receptors called ER -alpha and ER -beta (Venkov et al 1996, Iafrati et al 1997). ER alpha and ER beta are encoded by different genes and act as lig and dependant transcription factors (Green et al 1986). In mice, ER alpha and ER beta are both active (Walker and Korach 2004).

Human EPC's express ER alpha but not ER beta (Foresta et al 2007). In humans, estrogen receptor alpha activity mediates the response of estrogen on blood vessel walls including the acceleration of re-endothelialization and increased release of endothelial nitric oxide (Hamada et al 2006). Estrogen receptor beta is involved in gender differences in the protection from cardiovascular disease (Zhu et al 2002). Nitric oxide is a fat soluble compound released by vascular endothelial cells in response to a variety of stimuli (Petrofsky et al 2007a). Activation of estrogen receptors, by increasing the release of nitric oxide, induces vasodilation. This vasodilation is the result of nitric oxide increasing the formation of cyclic GMP in the surrounding smooth muscle (Petrofsky et al 2007a). This in turn decreases calcium permeability in vascular smooth muscle and hyperpolarizes the membrane by increasing potassium permeability (Petrofsky et al 2007b).

The exact signaling pathway associated with estrogen increasing levels of EPC's (Iwakura et al 2003, Strehlow et al 2003) is not known. Several studies indicate that the activation of PI3k/akt pathways may be involved (Assmus et al 2003, Dimmler et al 20, Carmen and Dimmeler 2008). Thus, if PI3k/akt is activated, this in turn would be one pathway activating nitric oxide synthetase (Carmen and Dimmeler 2004).

Because of the direct effect of estrogen on vascular genesis and angiogenesis through VEG-F (Carmen and Dimmeler 2004) estrogen in the circulation is also associated, in some models, with an increase in wound healing. Thus, even in males, organs such as the penis have been shown, in animal models, to have estrogen receptors (Crescioli et al. 2003, Dietrich et al 2004, Goyal et al 2007) and show increased healing from injury in response to estrogen (Mowa et al 2008). Part of the process is increased immune reactivity of VEGF in estrogen treated rats (Nissen et al 1998).

The evidence for the role of nitric oxide modulation in response to estrogen is derived in part from studies on pulmonary arterial vasoconstriction (Lahm et al 2008). Both endogenous and exogenous estrogens have been shown to decrease pulmonary arterial vasoconstriction under normoxic and hypoxic conditions (English et al 2001, Lahm et al 2008, Lahm et al 2007). This is not surprising since acute and chronic hypoxic pulmonary hypertension is less common and less pronounced in females than males (Lahm et al 2008, McLaughlin and McGoon 2006; Rabinovich et al 1981). This is also true in the systemic circulation. Both estrogen alpha and beta receptors have been demonstrated to mediate vasodilator effects of estrogen (Pare et al 2002; Zhu et al 2002).

There has been some controversy on whether the estrogen alpha or beta receptors are responsible in the systemic circulation for modulation of nitric oxide (Chambliss et al 2002; Chen et al 1999; Hisamoto et al 2001). In a recent study, it was shown that both the alpha and beta receptor were responsible for decreasing vasoconstriction through a nitric oxide dependant vasodilitory mechanism (Lahm 2008).

However, this response may be dose dependant. For example, Charkoudian et al (Charkoudian et al 1999a) demonstrated that cutaneous vasodilatation to local warming was increased when young women were taking oral contraceptives. In men, testosterone may inhibit nitric oxide dependant vasodilatation (Karakitsos et al 2006), a completely opposite effect. When small doses (less than those used in a birth control pill) of both testosterone and estrogen were given to a group of subjects during local warming,(Sokolnicki et al 2007) there was no effect of either estrogen or testosterone in changing the vasodilator response to local warming. Thus, this effect might be dose related. However, a large difference should be noted between this study and previous studies. In young men and women, testosterone reduced the blood flow response to local heat, whereas estrogen increased the blood flow response to local heat (Brooks et al 1997, Charkoudian 1999a).

However, in the recent study by Charkoudian et al (Sokolnicki et al 2007) older individuals were examined and this response was not seen. Thus, ageing may have an effect altering the estrogen receptor response of vascular endothelial cells. It is well established that ageing causes a decrease in the cutaneous vasodilator response (Kenney et al 1997, Martin et al 1995). This is also believed to be mediated, in part, through a diminished production or bioavailability of nitric oxide with ageing (Kenney et al 1997, Martin et al 1995). The diminished response to estrogen (Brooks et al 1997, Charkoudian 1999a) and testosterone (Karakitsos et al 2006) in older individuals may be due to the fact that the estrogen response may be mediated through defective nitric oxide transduction associated with age (see age below). There is no evidence that estrogen receptors as well as testosterone receptors are damaged with ageing. This is further complicated by diabetes. In people with diabetes, there is also damage to the nitric oxide pathway in vascular endothelial cells (Sang et al 2001).

It is not surprising, then, that estrogen has little to or no effect on endothelial dysfunction in postmenopausal women with diabetes. Here, ageing and diabetes both interact with potential pathways involved which are the same as those to normal estrogen alpha and beta receptors on vascular endothelial cells. Thus, the greatest effect of estrogen on blood flow is in younger women.

- **The influence of diabetes on skin circulation**

Both Type 1 and Type 2 Diabetes have similar effects on the autonomic nervous system. Although Type 1 diabetes, sometimes called juvenile diabetes, is an autoimmune disease, high glucose in the plasma still causes damage to the autonomic nervous system (Lacigova et al 2009; Comi et al 1986). Type 2 diabetes, sometimes called metabolic syndrome, has as its cause increase resistance of cells (including vascular endothelial cells and smooth muscle cells) to insulin (Vinik et al 2003; Maloney-Hinds et al 2009; Petrofsky et al 2008d; McLellan et al 2008).

In type 2 diabetes, hyperinsulinemia is common since the pancreas must overproduce insulin to compensate for resistance for the cell to the effect of insulin (Zhang et al 2008). In type 2 diabetes, the defect is not in the insulin receptor itself but in the transduction of the insulin receptor into an effect through the activation of phosphatidylinositol 3-kinase in the cells (Bulhak et al 2009) is impaired. Thus, in type 2 diabetes, insulin levels can rise to the point where the pancreas eventually is unable to continue producing insulin in pancreatic beta cells fail (McLellan et al 2008; Maloney-Hinds et al 2008; Petrofsky et al 2008d).

It is easy to understand how impaired production of phosphatidylinositol 3-kinase and the inherent shift in the metabolism in the cell to lipid metabolism in type 2 diabetes from carbohydrate metabolism could damage the cell (Vinik et al 2003). The common denominator with type 1 and type 2 diabetes in causing damage to vascular endothelial cells is twofold, high average glucose concentrations in the blood and, even more damage due to high peaks in glucose in the blood (Alemzadeh et al 2005).

It was once felt that the average level of glucose through in the body over 24 hours (as assessed by HbA1c) was the best predictor of autonomic nervous system damage and damage to the blood vessels and nerves associated with diabetes. However, recent studies have shown that more important than the average concentration of glucose in the blood or the variations in glucose that occur throughout the day, especially pre and postprandial (Peter et al 2009). Large spikes in glucose after a highcarbohydrate meal can do immediate damage to the autonomic nervous system. It has been reported that with hypoglycemic episodes or hyperglycemic episodes, the autonomic nervous system can go into shock for an excess of 24 hrs and not function properly (Peter et al 2009).

Because vascular endothelial cells in the autonomic nervous system are highly susceptible to high glycemic concentrations in the blood glucose, damage to these cells occurs in both type 1 and type 2 diabetes before the clinical diagnosis of these both types of diabetes (Vinik et al 2003; Petrofsky et al 2007d; Petrofsky et al 2007e; Lawson and Petrofsky 2007; Petrofsky et al 2006a). Thus, young children and adults, at the time of diagnosis of diabetes, already have autonomic damage and impairment in blood flow response in tissue (Vinik et al 2003).

In terms of the blood vessels of the skin, the damage is twofold. Damage of the sympathetic ganglia has been noted in type 2 diabetes (Northam et al 2009). This does not seem to impair vasoconstriction; however, the ability of the vascular smooth muscle to vasodilate is impaired with type 2 and type 1 diabetes (Vinik et al 2003; Petrofsky et al 2008d; McLellan et al 2008; Maloney-Hinds et al 2008). Damage to the parasympathetic and sympathetic nervous systems are quantified clinically by changes in heart rate variability (Vinik et al 2003; Niakan et al 1986; Hume et al 1986; Murray et al 1990; Langer et al 1991). Normally, vasomotor rhythm in the sympathetic and parasympathetic system causes the heart rate to vary continuously on a breath by breath and minute by minute basis (Vinik et al 2003). These different variations in heart rate can be seen by analysis of the EKG. As diabetes progresses, heart rate variability is less and less such that finally, sympathetic damage and parasympathetic damage have occurred to the extent that there is very little variation in heart rate with exercise or even a change in body position (Vinik et al 2003).

At the level of the blood vessels in the skin, the reduction of the sympathetic vasodilator activity is most evident and limits the response to global heat and other physiological stressors such as emotions (McLellan et al 2008; Maloney-Hinds et al 2008; Petrofsky et al 2008f). But the most direct damage to the skin occurs in damage to the actual endothelial cells themselves. Damage to vascular endothelial cells takes two forms. First, there appears to be less bioavailability of nitric oxide. Some studies point to the fact that the enzyme nitric oxide synthetase or, TRPV-4 calcium channels are damaged by high glycemic levels in type 2 diabetes (Maloney-Hinds 2009; Petrofsky et al 2007c).

This would reduce the nitric oxide production to a given vasodilator stimulus in a vascular endothelial cells. Other studies show that in diabetes, there is a reduced bioavailability of Arginine, altering the ability of the endothelial cells to produce nitric oxide. Other studies show that once nitric oxide is produced, the high free radical concentration in the body associated with both obesity and diabetes bioconvert nitric oxide into peroxynitrate and thus reduce nitric oxide's bioavailability as a vasodilator (Potenza et al 2009; Woodman et al 2005; Vinik et al 2003). Probably all three mechanisms are present to various extents in diabetes in different populations.

The overall effect is less nitric oxide bioavailability with the overall effect of less production of cyclic GMP in vascular smooth muscle. Therefore, with vasodilation impaired, vasoconstrictor tone in the skin blood vessels predominates in people with diabetes. There are also, morphological changes in the endothelial cell muscle interphase seen in diabetes (Potenza et al 2009; Woodman et al 2005).

Normally, small cellular attachments (electro tonic connections) occur between endothelial cells and vascular smooth muscle (Woodman et al 2005). Thus when endothelial cells depolarize or hyperpolarize the electro tonic connection through gap junctions helps coordinate electrical activity between endothelial cells and the surrounding vascular smooth muscle (Woodman et al 2005). When vasodilator effectors bind to the endothelial membrane, the endothelial cell hyperpolarizes through an increase in potassium permeability. This increase in potassium permeability then causes hyperpolarization in vascular smooth muscle making it harder to develop action potentials and thus aiding in the process of vasodilation (de Wit et al 2008; Gupta et al 2008). In people with diabetes, these electro tonic connections are destroyed and part of the ability of the endothelial cell to relax vascular smooth muscle through hyperpolarization is also lost (Triggle et al 2003).

The overall effect is that the blood flow at rest is less in skin and people with diabetes (by almost 66% reduction) due to a predominant vasoconstriction, blood flow response to global and local heat is reduced and therapeutic modalities such as contrast baths, which normally cause a large increase in blood flow in the skin are ineffective in people with diabetes (Maloney-Hinds 2009 ; Petrofsky et al 2007; McLellan et al 2008; Maloney-Hinds et al 2008; Petrofsky et al 2008; Sokolnicki et al 2008; Kvandal et al 2006).

For example, after 4 minutes of vascular occlusion, there is a reactive hyperemia (upper curve). But in people with diabetes, both resting and post occlusion hyperemia is reduced (lower curve). The skin blood flow response to stressors such as electrical stimulation, when used clinically for wound healing or therapy is also diminished (AlMalty et al 2008b; Suh et al 2008) Since the skin circulation relies more on nitric oxide in older individuals as people with diabetes age, this condition worsens disproportionately. A good example is the effect of contrast baths.

- **Race, lifestyle, and endothelial function**

In recent years, numerous studies have shown that obesity (Yudkin et al 2000; Ford 1999; Yudkin et al 1999; Hak et al 1999; Weyer et al 2000; Fresta et al 2000), cigarette smoking (Antoniades et al 2008), and race (Mata-Greenwood and Chen 2008) are associated with chronic inflammation and changes in vascular endothelial cells that are associated with cardiovascular disease. For example, adipose tissue expresses a variety of cytokines including IL-6, TNF alpha (Yudkin et al 2000; Yudkin et al 1999; Hak et al 1999; Weyer et al 2000; Fresta et al 2000) which increases the production of C Reactive Protein (CRP) (Heinrich et al 1990). These inflammatory processes are involved in early stages of atherogenesis (Hanson et al 1989; Yokota and Hanson 1995) which can result in endothelial cell damage as well as damage to other cells in the body and lead to the pathogenesis of insulin resistance (Pickup et al 1997; Pickup and Crock 1998; Fernandez-Real 1999).

IL-6 and TNF alpha cause the release of endothelial adhesion molecules and impair insulin action by interfering with the insulin signaling cascade (Van der Poll et al 1992 Hotamisligil et al 1994). CRP, elevated due to inflammatory cytokines, cause impaired endothelium dependant vasodilatation by interfering with either endothelial nitric oxide synthetase (ENOS) or endothelial nitric oxide bioavailability (Fichtlscherer et al 2000). Endothelial cells, especially those in the capillaries, have been shown to predict cardiovascular events (Jager et al 1999; Jager et al 2000; Ridker et al 1998). And vascular endothelial damage as evidence from markers such as E-selectin, and soluble vascular adhesion molecule (SVCAM-1) are highly predictive of damage to these endothelial cells and damage to the circulation in the skin and other organs (Albelda et al 1994; O'Brien et al 1996; Gearing and Newman 1993; Jager et al 2000; Hwang et al 1997).

Environmental factors such as smoking are also key to causing damage to vascular endothelial cells (Thomas et al 2008). Smoking is considered a major risk factor for atherogenesis and vascular diseases (Surgeon General 1990; Lam et al 1997). Tobacco smoke contains more than 4,000 chemicals many of which can lead to pathological changes in the endothelial cells of the vascular system (Davis et al 1985). Oxygen free radicals from tobacco smoking increase cellular oxidation and can impair bioavailability of nitric oxide (Davis et al 1985). These radicals oxidize nitric oxide to chemicals such as peroxynitrate, a superoxide, which can further damage tissue by lipid peroxidation of membranes (Thomas et al 2008).

Smoking has also been reported to increase sympathetic nerve activity and thus contributing to vascular tone in overriding vasodilators released from the vascular endothelium (Krkiewicz et al 1998). Smoking also increases levels of protein fibrinogen thus having prothrombotic effects (Lam et al 1999). Thus, in addition to inhibition vasodilation of arteries, smoking has multiple effects on the health of vascular endothelial cells (Woo et al 1997; Woo et al 2000; yip et al 2007; Vapaatalo and Mervaala 2001).

The whole situation becomes more complex when considering race into. Most data on the effect of race on vasodilation has been done by measuring vascular reactivity to various challenges such as vascular occlusion (Mata-Greenwood and Chen 2008). The test measures the effect of ischemia on blood flow in blood vessels in the skin, by using a laser Doppler imager, or using an ultrasound on larger arteries such as the brachial artery (Mata-Greenwood and Chen 2008). However, tests of vascular function also include the use of agonists of sympathetic activity such as acetylcholine or methylcholine can be used to activate muscarinic receptors on vascular endothelial cells which then leads to an increase in intracellular calcium and therefore up regulation of ENOS and release of nitric oxide (Furchgott and Zawadzki 1980; Wang et al 1994). Bradykinin which activates ENOS can also be used (Harris et al 2001).

A recent review article summarized many of the differences associates with race seen in nitric oxide dependant vasodilatation (Mata-Greenwood and Chen 2008). Briefly, Afro-Americans show a decreased vasodilitory response to methylcholine and albuterol in spite of the fact they were healthy and young (Lteif et al 2005; Kalra et al 2005; Radomski et al 1987). With a decrease of vasodilitory response to stress, it is not surprising that, withinafro Americans, 30 and 20 % of deaths in men and women respectively are caused by hypertension (Lapu-Bula and Ofili 2007; Hajjar and Kotchen 2003). Thus, a decrease in nitric oxidedependant vasodilatation is very evident in this population (Bragulat et al 2001). There is also an increase incidence of asthma (McDaniel et al 2006) and type 2 diabetes associated with insulin resistance (McBean et al 2004; Ferdinand and Clark 2004).

Asians and Indians are comparable and have a higher incidence of both type 2 diabetes and impaired vascular response to vasodilators (McKeigue et al 1991; Balarajan et al 1991). In comparing Europeans of African descent to Americans of African descent, the nitric oxide dysfunction in vascular endothelial cells is even greater (Kahn et al 2002; An drone et al 2006). Thus other factors are involved other than racial origin such as environmental influencescomparing Africans of European vs. American origin. However, both groups did exhibit greater endothelial dysfunction than Caucasians. A few studies have examined the mechanism by which Afro Americans and European Americans have differences in endothelial dependant vasodilatation. ENOS, from Afro Americans, is actually more active than ENOS from European Americans in some studies (Kalinowski et al 2004; Mason et al).

However, while ENOS is more active in afro Americans, production of reactive oxygen species is greater than that found in European Caucasians. This causes nitric oxide to be bioconverted to peroxynitrate and reduces nitric oxide bioavailability (Kalinowski et al 2004; Mason et al). Thus nitric oxide bioavailability is lower, although ENOS activity is higher in afro Americans. Other races have gene polymorphisms that also skin blood flow. Asians, for example, genetically have a deficiency in the "thrifty gene". The thrifty gene codes the production of peroxisome proliferator activated receptor (PPAR), a nuclear subtransmitter that up regulates carbohydrate metabolism in the cell. This single nucleotide polymorphism has been reported to have a preventive role in the development of diabetes by decreasing insulin resistance (Tai et al 2004; Radha et al 2006; Hara et al 2002). The defect in the gene is Asians may be responsible for the fact that Asians are not able to tolerate high fat food. South Asian men have been shown to have lower brachial artery dilation to occlusion, lower vasodilitory response to acetylcholine, higher level of insulin resistance, and higher CRP compared to Caucasian men of a similar age and anthropometric measurements (Murphy et al 2007).

Thus, by altering carbohydrate metabolism in Asians due to the thrifty gene difference, ingestion of a high fat meal, which normally increases free fatty acid concentration in the blood, can affect nitric oxide production (Tsai et al 2004; Bae et al 2001; Tripathy et al 2003). Normally an increase in plasma free fatty acid concentration after ingestion of a high fat meal is associated with induction of pro inflammatory cytokines (Nappo et al 2002) and reactive oxygen species within the vascular walls (Kalinowski et al 2002; Wallenstein et al 1980). This then causes an increase in activation of nuclear factor kappa beta as well as generation of reactive oxygen species (Tripathy et al 2003). These super oxides can bind with nitric oxide producing peroxy nitrate and other superoxides reducing the bioavailability of nitric oxide after a high fat meal (Nappo et al 2002; Tripathy et al 2003; Sears et al 2002). In addition, free fatty acids can induce protein kinase C which inhibits phosphotinol 3 kinase thereby inhibiting the activity and activation of endothelial nitric oxide synthetase (Bakker et al 2008; Dresner et al 1999; Griffin et al 1999).

Asians, due to genetic differences, are more susceptible to vascular endothelial impairment. But even within the Asian population, environmental influence is also important. For example, westernization of lifestyles in Japan and for native Japanese men who have moved to the United States, there is an increase in cardiovascular disease and vascular endothelial dysfunction (Watanabe et al 2004).

In other minority populations within the United States such as Pima Indians (Krakoff et al 2003) endothelial dysfunction and the incidence of diabetes is also much higher. However, genesis of this endothelial dysfunction in populations such as Native Americans is poorly understood (Weyer et al 2002). What is known is that markers of endothelial dysfunction such as insulin resistance and low-grade inflammation (elevated CRP and other cytokines) are common in Native Americans such as Pima Indians (Weyer et al 2002). Other markers of endothelial dysfunction such as E-selectin and Von Willebrand factor were also elevated in pima Indians as well as soluble intracellular adhesion molecule -1 (Sicam -1) compared to Caucasians living in similar areas. These same markers of endothelial dysfunction have been reported in Koreans as well (Kim et al 2008). Further, in Asians, the increase incidence in cigarette smoking increases free radicals not only blocking the release of nitric oxide, but the damage extends into vascular smooth muscle with free radical oxidation of many pathways of vascular smooth muscle (Antoniades et al 2008). Even children exposed to passive smoking show increase in oxidative markers (Kosecik et al 2005). The mechanism of vascular smooth muscle damage of oxidative stress is not known (Antoniades et al 2008).

Some modifications of endothelial nitric oxide synthetase are not necessarily bad. For example, in Sherpa's (Droma et al 2006) modification in nitric oxide metabolism allows for greater vasodilatation in systemic and pulmonary arteries during hypoxia. Thus, this population is able to tolerate high altitude much better than other individuals in other races due to a specific polymorphism in endothelial nitric oxide synthetase (Droma et al 2006).

This section by no means covers all races. For example, a recent study on gene polymorphisms and endogenous nitric oxide synthetase gene on chromosome 7q35 through 36 was accomplished on north and south Indian populations (Periaswamy et al 2008). This study described an endogenous nitric oxide synthetase gene polymorphism associated with an impaired production of nitric oxide in response to stress which then resulted in more susceptibility to endothelial dysfunction, hypertension and diabetes (Periaswamy et al 2008). Studies have been both accomplished on both south Indian populations (Shoji et al 2000; Kato et al 1999; Benjafield and Morris 2000) and northern Indian populations (Srivastava et al 2008; Tamil People 2008).

- **Ageing**

Normally, aging results in the natural senescence of multiple organ systems including the kidney (Fagard et al 1993), the autonomic nervous system (Cybulski and Niewiadomski 2003), and the heart (Rzeczuch et al 2003). While numerous mechanisms are involved in agerelated changes in the body, one important factor contributing to decreased function is a reduction in nitric oxide production (a potent vasodilator) in tissues (Stadler et al 2003). In addition, there is a reduction in beta adrenergic receptor sensitivity associated with the aging process (Schutzer and Mader 2003), reducing the ability of the sympathetic nervous system to respond to stress.

Thus ageing principally affects three areas associated with circulatory control. The first of these is the vascular endothelial cell itself. The next is control of the sympathetic nervous system as it alters the control of the peripheral circulation. Finally, there is a thinning of the dermal layer of the skin (Petrofsky 2008d; Petrofsky 2008e). Reduced endothelial function appears to occur gradually throughout life, accelerating in the later years. Disorders such as diabetes accelerate endothelial dysfunction with age (Petrofsky et al 2004). Since diabetes accelerates with ageing, the interaction of age and diabetes becomes important clinically.

As people age, most studies show a small decrease in blood pressure and loss in heart rate variability during orthostatic stress (Shi et al 2001; Siebert et al 2004; Konrady et al 2001). This would seem to indicate aging has only a small effect on the autonomic nervous system. However, if additional stressors are placed on the autonomic nervous system, such as heat exposure during orthostatic stress, the reduction in blood pressure with age is much more pronounced (Scremin et al 2004). While there is a general reduction in autonomic function with ageing (Ray and Monahan 2002), it has been established that there is also a decrease in baroreceptor sensitivity with aging (Gribbin 1971; Guyton and Harris 1951), masking sudden changes in body position. The common denominator in all of the age related changes in organ function is damage to the microcirculation.

While there is no documented reduction in the ability of the blood vessels to vasoconstrict, there is a marked reduction in the ability of vessels to vasodilate with age (Franzoni et al 2004). Therefore, vasoconstrictor tone predominates and blood flow at rest and during an autonomic stress is reduced (Franzoni et al 2004). The mechanism of the loss in vasodilatation appears to be twofold. First, there is a reduction in the release of nitric oxide, a vasodilator, from skin blood vessels associated with the aging process (Franzoni et al 2004). Second, reducing sympathetic activity further, beta adrenergic receptor sensitivity is also reduced with ageing due to structural changes in the receptor making it insensitive to catecholamines (Schutzer and Mader 2003). Finally, aging also reduces the sensitivity of the parasympathetic nervous system.

- **Interaction between Age and Diabetes**

Diabetes, like age, is associated with damage to the autonomic nervous system (Accurso et al 2001). Recent studies show that damage to autonomic nerves can occur prior to any clinical symptoms of diabetes causing orthostatic intolerance (Sagliocco et al 1999). Damage to the parasympathetic nervous system results in the loss in the control of heart rate, especially during orthostatic stress (Ewing et al 1991). The damage is usually found both at the autonomic ganglia and also at the peripheral nerve endings where microcirculation is critical. During orthostatic challenge, when subjects are exposed to a thermally neutral environment, it has been estimated that 25% of diabetic patients show a drop of 20 mmHg (0.266 kPa) or more in mean blood pressure (Agrawal 1999; Ewing and Clarke 1986). However, when multiple autonomic stressors are added, such as increasing room temperature, the systolic blood pressure falls in almost all patients with diabetes (Petrofsky et al 2003a; Petrofsky et al 2003b).

The mechanism in diabetes appears to be an inability to vasodilate blood vessels (Stansberry 1999). Like aging, the damage appears to be twofold. First, damage of the ability of the autonomic nerves to generate impulses due to ganglionic damage and second an inability to release adequate nitric oxide associated with diabetes (Hsueh and Law 1998). These factors affect both arterial and venous circulations (Winer Sowers 2003).

Thus diabetes seems to cause similar damage to the autonomic nervous system and endothelial cell function as normally occurs with aging. For this reason, diabetes has been said to increase the aging process by increasing the severity of the loss of autonomic function. Neuronal damage can be so pronounced as to cause lesions of the spinal cord (Varsik et al 2001).

In addition to nerve and circulatory damage, another factor also seems to come into play with both ageing and diabetes. This is thickness of the dermal layer of the skin. Ageing has been associated with a reduction in skin blood flow and numerous changes in the structure of the skin including changes in skin collagen, skin thickness, and the response of the skin vasculature to local and global heat stress (Branchet et al 1990; Puig et al 1990). For example, with both diabetes and age, resting blood flow is less. However, at the same age, diabetes causes a greater reduction in blood flow than age alone. The administration of Rosiglitazone for 6 months did reverse the diabetes effect on resting and post occlusion blood flows, but not the age effects, pointing to different mechanisms for endothelial damage.

Recent studies verify that skin dermal layer thickness decreases with ageing (Petrofsky et al 2008d; Petrofsky et al 2008e). The thinner skin in older people has been reported to be due to a thickening in the stratus corneum and a thinning in the dermal layer. A thinning in the dermal layer implies less vasculature in the skin in older rather than younger people. This was also true in people with diabetes. Thinner skin should make the skin more susceptible to damage such as burns and injuries and, as is the case for people with diabetes, make the skin harder to heal. The subcutaneous fat layer is also reduced in thickness with ageing (Petrofsky et al 2008e; Puig et al 1990; Schwartz et al 1990; Fu and Fung 1995).

This may be critical for the foot especially due to even greater thinning in people with diabetes on the foot since the reduction in the thickness of foot padding would make the foot more susceptible to lesions during gait. When added to the thinner dermal layer in the skin, this would make the skin even harder to heal. It has been assumed that the reduction in blood flow with ageing and diabetes is solely due to impairment in nitric oxide synthesis, a vascular endothelial mediator of vascular smooth muscle dilatation (Petrofsky et al 2006b; Petrofsky et al 2005a; Petrofsky et al 2007d). But thinner skin would certainly mean less blood vessel density and also account for some of the reduction in skin blood flow. Making matters worse, the high correlation between subcutaneous fat and BMI and the greater BMI in the subjects with diabetes would imply that their fat layer should even be thinner if they had normal weight. Thus someone with diabetes, but thin, would even be more susceptible to foot injuries during gait.

When these data are coupled with the effects of race and gender as described above. The status of blood vessels in human populations is complex and altered by many factors, let alone factors not discussed here that have taken recent interest such as pollutants in the air and water, both of which impair endothelial vascular function. Recent studies show that particulate matter form diesel engines can activate the JNK pathway and damage endothelial function (Li et al 2008, Nuckles et al 2008). This same effect on ENOS pathways is true of cigarette smoke (Fira-Mladinescu et al 2008) and air pollution in general (O'toole et al 2008). Thus many factors alter endothelial function.

References

Accurso V, Shamsuzzaman AS, Somers VK: Rhythms, rhymes, and reasons--spectral oscillations in neural cardiovascular control. Auton Neurosci, 2001; 20(90):41-6

Agner , T., Damm, P. & Skouby, S. (1991). Menstrual cycle and skin reactivity. Journal of the American Academy of Dermatology, 24, 566-570.

Aguilera-Saez, J., Binimelis, M. M., Collado, J. M., Dos Santos, B. P., Garcia, V., Ruiz-Castilla, M., . . . Barret, J. P. (2016). Electrical burns in times of economic crisis: A new epidemiologic profile. Burns. doi:10.1016/j.burns.2016.06.016

Agrawal A, Saran R, Khanna R: Management of orthostatic hypotension from autonomic dysfunction in diabetics on peritoneal dialysis. Perit Dial Int, 1999; 19:415-7

Albelda, S. M., C. W. Smith, et al. (1994). "Adhesion molecules and inflammatory injury." FASEB J 8(8): 504-12.

Alderton, W. K., C. E. Cooper, et al. (2001). "Nitric oxide synthases: structure, function and inhibition." Biochem J 357(Pt 3): 593-615.

Alemzadeh, R., P. Palma-Sisto, et al. (2005). "Continuous subcutaneous insulin infusion and multiple dose of insulin regimen display similar patterns of blood glucose excursions in pediatric type 1 diabetes." Diabetes Technol Ther 7(4): 587-96.

AlMalty AM, Petrofsky J. The effect of stimulation on a normal skin blood flow in active young and older adults. Med Sci Monit. 2007 April;13(4): CR147-55.

Al Malty, Petrofsky, J. A. & Suh, H.J. (2007). Isometric endurance, body and skin temperature and limb and skin blood flow during the menstrual cycle. Medical science monitor,13(3), cr 111-cr 117.

AlMalty A, Petrofsky J, Akhavan S. (2008a). "Aging in women: The effect of menopause on skin blood flow and the response to electrical stimulation." Physical &Occupational Ther in Ger. 1-21.

AlMalty, A., Petrofsky, J.S., Gunda, S., Prowse, M. (2008b). Relationship between Multiple Stimuli and the Response of Vascular Endothelial Cells submitted Saudi J Rehabilitation

Alves, E., Angrisani, A., & Santiago, M. (2009). The use of extracorporeal shock waves in the treatment of osteonecrosis of the femoral head: a systematic review. *Clin Rheumatol. 28*, 1247–1251.

Anderson, M. A. a. P., G.P. (2012). Foundations of Athletic Training: Prevention, Assessment, and Management (5th ed.): Wolters Kluwer Health/Lippincott Williams & Wilkins.

Androne, A. S., K. Hryniewicz, et al. (2006). "Comparison of metabolic vasodilation in response to exercise and ischemia and endothelium-dependent flow-mediated dilation in African-American versus non-African-American patients with chronic heart failure." Am J Cardiol 97(5): 685-9.

Antoniades, C., D. Tousoulis, et al. (2008). "Smoking in Asians: it doesn't stop at vascular endothelium." Int J Cardiol 128(2): 151-3.

Arnal JF et al Estrogens in vascular biology and disease: where do we stand today? Curr Op Lipidol 18 (2007), pp.554-560.

Aruga, T., & Miyake, Y. (2012). [Pathophysiology of heat illness]. Nihon Rinsho, 70(6), 940-946.

Asahara, T., T. Murohara, et al. (1997). "Isolation of putative progenitor endothelial cells for angiogenesis." Science 275(5302): 964-7.

Assmus, B., C. Urbich, et al. (2003). "HMG-CoA reductase inhibitors reduce senescence and increase proliferation of endothelial progenitor cells via regulation of cell cycle regulatory genes." Circ Res 92(9): 1049-55.

Bae, J. H., E. Bassenge, et al. (2001). "Postprandial hypertriglyceridemia impairs endothelial function by enhanced oxidant stress." Atherosclerosis 155(2): 517-23.

Bakker, W., P. Sipkema, et al. (2008). "Protein kinase C theta activation induces insulin-mediated constriction of muscle resistance arteries." Diabetes 57(3): 706-13.

Balarajan, R. (1991). "Ethnic differences in mortality from ischaemic heart disease and cerebrovascular disease in England and Wales." BMJ 302(6776): 560-4.

Benjafield, A. V. and B. J. Morris (2000). "Association analyses of endothelial nitric oxide synthase gene polymorphisms in essential hypertension." Am J Hypertens 13(9): 994-8.

Bennett, L. A., J. M. Johnson, et al. (2003). "Evidence for a role for vasoactive intestinal peptide in active vasodilatation in the cutaneous vasculature of humans." J Physiol 552(Pt 1): 223-32.

Bern R.M.,Levey M.N., Koeppen, B.M & Stanton B.A (2004) , The microcirculation and lymphatic. In : Physiology, 5th edition, ch.20, PP.383-387. Mosby

Bigley, G. K. (1990). Sensation. In H. K. Walker, W. D. Hall, & J. W. Hurst (Eds.), Clinical Methods: The History, Physical, and Laboratory Examinations (3rd ed.). Boston.

Blair, D. A., W. E. Glover, et al. (1959). "The abolition of reactive and post-exercise hyperaemia in the forearm by temporary restriction of arterial inflow." J Physiol 148: 648-58.

Block, S. S. (2001). *Disinfection, Sterilization, and Preservation.* Philadelphia: Lippincott Williams & Wilkins.

Boucaud, A. (2004). Trends in the use of ultrasound-mediated transdermal drug delivery. *Drug Discov Today. 9*, 827–828.

Bradley, E., A. Law, et al. (2003). "Effects of varying impulse number on cotransmitter contributions to sympathetic vasoconstriction in rat tail artery." Am J Physiol Heart Circ Physiol 284(6): H2007-14.

Bragulat, E., A. de la Sierra, et al. (2001). "Endothelial dysfunction in salt-sensitive essential hypertension." Hypertension 37(2 Part 2): 444-8.

Branchet MC, Boisnic S, Frances C, Robert A .Skin thickness changes in normal aging skin. Gerontology.1990;36(1):28-35.

Brock Symons, T., Clasey, J. L., Gater, D. R., & Yates, J. W. (2004). Effects of deep heat as a preventative mechanism on delayed onset muscle soreness. J Strength Cond Res, 18(1), 155-161.

Brooks, E. M., A. L. Morgan, et al. (1997). "Chronic hormone replacement therapy alters thermoregulatory and vasomotor function in postmenopausal women." J Appl Physiol 83(2): 477-84.

Brucker, J. B., Knight, K. L., Rubley, M. D., & Draper, D. O. (2005). An 18-day stretching regimen, with or without pulsed, shortwave diathermy, and ankle dorsiflexion after 3 weeks. J Athl Train, 40(4), 276-280.

Brunner, H., J. R. Cockcroft, et al. (2005). "Endothelial function and dysfunction. Part II: Association with cardiovascular risk factors and diseases. A statement by the Working Group on Endothelins and Endothelial Factors of the European Society of Hypertension." J Hypertens 23(2): 233-46.

Bungum, L., Kvernebo, K., Oian, P. & Maltau, J. (1996). Laser Doppler recorded reactive hyperaemia in the forearm skin during the menstrual cycle. British journal of Obstetrics &Gynaecology, 103, 70-75

Butt, E., M. Bernhardt, et al. (2000). "Endothelial nitric-oxide synthase (type III) is activated and becomes calcium independent upon phosphorylation by cyclic nucleotide-dependent protein kinases." J Biol Chem 275(7): 5179-87.

Calleja-Agius J, Muscat-Baron Y, Brincat MP. Skin aging. Menopause Int.2007 Jun;13(2):60-4

Cankar, K. Finderle, Z. Strucl, M. (2000). Gender difference in cutaneous laser Doppler flow response to local direct on contra-lateral cooling. Journal of vascular research, 37,183-188.

Carmen, J., Roeder, B., Nelson, J., Beckstead, B., Runyan, C., Schaalje, G., et al. (2004). Ultrasonically enhanced vancomycin activity against Staphylococcus epidermidis biofilms in vivo. *Journal of biomaterials applications 18 (4)*, 237–45.

Carmen U, Dimmeler S. (2004) Endothelial Progenitor Cells Characterization and Role in Vascular Biology. Circulation Research 344-353.

Cetin, N., Aytar, A., Atalay, A., & Akman, M. N. (2008). Comparing hot pack, short-wave diathermy, ultrasound, and TENS on isokinetic strength, pain, and functional status of women with osteoarthritic knees: a single-blind, randomized, controlled trial. Am J Phys Med Rehabil, 87(6), 443-451. doi:10.1097/PHM.0b013e318174e467

Ceradini, D. J., A. R. Kulkarni, et al. (2004). "Progenitor cell trafficking is regulated by hypoxic gradients through HIF-1 induction of SDF-1." Nat Med 10(8): 858-64.

Chambliss, K. L., I. S. Yuhanna, et al. (2002). "ERbeta has nongenomic action in caveolae." Mol Endocrinol 16(5): 938-46.

Chan NN, Valance P, Colhoum HM. Nitric oxide and vascular responses in type I diabetes. Diabetologia. 43: 137-147, 2000.

Chapman, B. L., Liebert, R. B., Lininger, M. R., & Groth, J. J. (2007). An introduction to physical therapy modalities. Adolesc Med State Art Rev, 18(1), 11-23, vii-viii.

Charalambos Antoniades, Dimitris Tousoulis,Christodoulos Stefanadis, 2007; Smoking in Asians: It doesn't stop at vascular endothelium.international jo cardiology 128 (2008) 151-153.

Charasuraisin, C, Berk, L, Petrofsky, JS, Montgomery, S., Shavlik, D., Hubbard, R (2008) Can a Single High-Fat Meal Impair Endothelial and Autonomic Function?, #2008-LB-4930-Diabetes

Charkoudian, N., D. P. Stephens, et al. (1999a). "Influence of female reproductive hormones on local thermal control of skin blood flow." J Appl Physiol 87(5): 1719-23.

Charkoudian, N. Johnson, J,(1999b). Reflex control of cutaneous vasoconstrictor system is reset by exogenous female reproductive hormones. J Appl Physiol 87:381-385.

Charkoudian, N. Johnson, J,(1999c). Altered reflex control of cutaneous circulation by female sex steroid is independent of prostaglandins. The American journal of physiology, 276, H1634-H1640.

Charkoudian N. (2003). Skin blood flow in adult human thermogregulation; how it works, when it does no tand why. Mayo Clinic Proceedings, 78, 603-612.

Charkoudian, N.,Joyner, M. J.(2004) Physiologic considerations for exercise performance in women. Clin Chest Med. (2004) Jun;25(2):247-55.

Chen, Z., I. S. Yuhanna, et al. (1999). "Estrogen receptor alpha mediates the nongenomic activation of endothelial nitric oxide synthase by estrogen." J Clin Invest 103(3): 401-6.

Chen, Z. P., K. I. Mitchelhill, et al. (1999). "AMP-activated protein kinase phosphorylation of endothelial NO synthase." FEBS Lett 443(3): 285-9.

Collins, K. (2005). Anatomy Academy: Nervous System, Senses and Glands, Book 3: Prufrock Press Inc.

Comi, G., N. Canal, et al. (1986). "Peripheral nerve abnormalities in newly-diagnosed diabetic children." Acta Diabetol Lat 23(1): 69-75.

Coyle EF, Montain SJ: Benefits of fluid replacement with carbohydrate during exercise. Med Sci Sports Exerc, 1992, 24:S324-30

Crescioli, C., M. Maggi, et al. (2003). "Expression of functional estrogen receptors in human fetal male external genitalia." J Clin Endocrinol Metab 88(4): 1815-24.

Cybulski G, Niewiadomski W: Influence of age on the immediate heart rate response to the active orthostatic test. J Physiol Pharmacol 2003, 54:65-80.

Davis, J. W., L. Shelton, et al. (1985). "Effects of tobacco and non-tobacco cigarette smoking on endothelium and platelets." Clin Pharmacol Ther 37(5): 529-33.

Dehghan, M., & Farahbod, F. (2014). The efficacy of thermotherapy and cryotherapy on pain relief in patients with acute low back pain, a clinical trial study. J Clin Diagn Res, 8(9), LC01-04. doi:10.7860/JCDR/2014/7404.4818

de la Torre JC,Aliev G,Inhibition of vascular nitric oxide after rat chronic brain hypoperfusion : spatial memory and immunocytochemical changes.J Cereb Blood Flow Metab 2005;25:663-672. (pubMed: 15703700)

de Wit, C., M. Boettcher, et al. (2008). "Signaling across myoendothelial gap junctions--fact or fiction?" Cell Commun Adhes 15(3): 231-45.

Dietrich, W., A. Haitel, et al. (2004). "Expression of estrogen receptors in human corpus cavernosum and male urethra." J Histochem Cytochem 52(3): 355-60.

Dietz, N. M., J. M. Rivera, et al. (1994). "Is nitric oxide involved in cutaneous vasodilation during body heating in humans?" J Appl Physiol 76(5): 2047-53.

Dimmeler, S., B. Assmus, et al. (1998). "Fluid shear stress stimulates phosphorylation of Akt in human endothelial cells: involvement in suppression of apoptosis." Circ Res 83(3): 334-41.

Dimmeler, S., I. Fleming, et al. (1999). "Activation of nitric oxide synthase in endothelial cells by Akt-dependent phosphorylation." Nature 399(6736): 601-5.

Dimmeler, S., A. Aicher, et al. (2001). "HMG-CoA reductase inhibitors (statins) increase endothelial progenitor cells via the PI 3-kinase/Akt pathway." J Clin Invest 108(3): 391-7.

Donnerer, J., R. Schuligoi, et al. (1993). "Upregulation, release and axonal transport of substance P and calcitonin gene-related peptide in adjuvant inflammation and regulatory function of nerve growth factor." Regul Pept 46(1-2): 150-4.

Draper, D. (2010). Induction cable diathermy and joint mobilization restore range of motion in a post-operative ACL patient. *Athl Ther Today 15(1)*, 36-38.

Dresner, A., D. Laurent, et al. (1999). "Effects of free fatty acids on glucose transport and IRS-1-associated phosphatidylinositol 3-kinase activity." J Clin Invest 103(2): 253-9.

Droma, Y., M. Hanaoka, et al. (2006). "Genetic contribution of the endothelial nitric oxide synthase gene to high altitude adaptation in sherpas." High Alt Med Biol 7(3): 209-20.

English, K. M., R. D. Jones, et al. (2001). "Gender differences in the vasomotor effects of different steroid hormones in rat pulmonary and coronary arteries." Horm Metab Res 33(11): 645-52.

Escoffre, J.-M., & Bouakaz, A. (2015). *Therapeutic Ultrasound.* Berlin: Springer.

Eugenia Mata-Greenwood,PhD,PharmD and Dong-Bao Chen,PhD. Racial Differences in nitric Oxide-Dependent Vasorelaxation. From the Department of Reproductive Medicine,University of Califona,San Diego.Reprod Sci.2008 January;15(1):9-25.

Ewing DJ, Clarke BF: Autonomic neuropathy: its diagnosis and prognosis. Clin Endocrinol Metab, 1986; 15:855-88

Ewing DJ, Boland O, Neilson JM, Cho CG, Clarke BF: Autonomic neuropathy, QT interval lengthening, and unexpected deaths in male diabetic patients. Diabetologia, 1991; 34:182-5

F. Xu, T. J. L., K.A. Seffen. (2008). Skin thermal pain modeling—A holistic method. Journal of Thermal Biology, 33(4), 223-237. doi:10.1016/j.jtherbio.2008.01.004

Fagard R, Thijs L, Amery A: Age and the Homodynamic Response to Posture and Exercise. Am J Geriatr Cardiol 1993, 2:23-40.

Farrell, D. M. and V. S. Bishop (1995). "Permissive role for nitric oxide in active thermoregulatory vasodilation in rabbit ear." Am J Physiol 269(5 Pt 2): H1613-8.

Fatemi, A. (2009). High-intensity focused ultrasound effectively reduces adipose tissue. *Semin Cutan Med Surg. 28*, 257–262.

Fernandez-Real JM,Ricard W. Insulin resistance and inflammation in an evolutionary perspective: the contribution of cytokine genotype/pnenotype to thriftiness. Diabetologia 1999;42:1367-74.

Ferdinand, K. C. and L. T. Clark (2004). "The epidemic of diabetes mellitus and the metabolic syndrome in African Americans." Rev Cardiovasc Med 5 Suppl 3: S28-33.

Festa, A., R. D'Agostino, Jr., et al. (2000). "Chronic subclinical inflammation as part of the insulin resistance syndrome: the Insulin Resistance Atherosclerosis Study (IRAS)." Circulation 102(1): 42-7.

Fichtlscherer S, Rosenberger G, Walter DH, Breuer S, Dimmeler S, Zeilher AM. Elevated C-reactive protein levels and impaired endothelial vasoreactivity in patients with coronary artery disease.Circulation 2000;102:1000-6.

Fira-Mladinescu O, Noveanu L, Ordodi V, Fira-Mladinescu C, Tudorache V, Mihalaş G. The effects of chronic exposure to cigarette smoke on vasomotor endothelial function of guinea pig pulmonary arteries Rev Med Chir Soc Med Nat Iasi. 2008 Jan-Mar;112(1):213-9.

Fitzgerald, J. E., Malik, M., & Ahmed, I. (2011). A single-blind controlled study of electrocautery and ultrasonic scalpel smoke plumes in laparoscopic surgery. *Surgical Endoscopy 26 (2)*, 337–42.

Foley, J., Little, J., & Vaezy, S. (2008). Effects of high-intensity focused ultrasound on nerve conduction. *Muscle Nerve. 37*, 241–250.

Ford, E. S. (1999). "Body mass index, diabetes, and C-reactive protein among U.S. adults." Diabetes Care 22(12): 1971-7.

Foresta, C., D. Zuccarello, et al. (2007). "Oestrogen stimulates endothelial progenitor cells via oestrogen receptor-alpha." Clin Endocrinol (Oxf) 67(4): 520-5.

Forstermann, U., E. I. Closs, et al. (1994). "Nitric oxide synthase isozymes. Characterization, purification, molecular cloning, and functions." Hypertension 23(6 Pt 2): 1121-31.

Forstermann, U., I. Gath, et al. (1995). "Isoforms of nitric oxide synthase. Properties, cellular distribution and expressional control." Biochem Pharmacol 50(9): 1321-32.

Fox, R. H. and O. G. Edholm (1963). "Nervous control of the cutaneous circulation." Br Med Bull 19: 110-4.

Franzoni F, Galetta F, Morizzo C et al: Effects of age and physical fitness on microcirculatory function. Clin Sci (Lond), 2004; 106(3):329-35

French, S. D., Cameron, M., Walker, B. F., Reggars, J. W., & Esterman, A. J. (2006). A Cochrane review of superficial heat or cold for low back pain. Spine (Phila Pa 1976), 31(9), 998-1006. doi:10.1097/01.brs.0000214881.10814.64

Fromy B, Abraham P, Aumet JL. Non-nociceptive capsaisin-sensitive nerve terminal stimulation allows for an original vasodilatory reflex in the human skin. Brain Res. 811: 166-168, 1998.

Fromy B, Merzeau S, Abrahan P, Saumet JL. Mechanisms of the cutaneous vasodilator response to local external pressure application in rate: involvement of the CGRP, neurokins, prostaglandins and NO. Br J Pharmacol. 2000;131:1161-11171.

Fu FH, Fung L. Distribution of subcutaneous fat and equations for predicting percent body fat from skinfold measurements: a comparison between Chinese females from two age cohorts. J Sports Med Phys Fitness. 1995 Sep;35(3):224-7.

Fulton, D., J. P. Gratton, et al. (1999). "Regulation of endothelium-derived nitric oxide production by the protein kinase Akt." Nature 399(6736): 597-601.

Fulton, D., J. P. Gratton, et al. (2001). "Post-translational control of endothelial nitric oxide synthase: why isn't calcium/calmodulin enough?" J Pharmacol Exp Ther 299(3): 818-24.

Furchgott, R. F. and J. V. Zawadzki (1980). "The obligatory role of endothelial cells in the relaxation of arterial smooth muscle by acetylcholine." Nature 288(5789): 373-6

Garry A, Sigaudo-Roussel D, Merzeau S, Odile D, S aumet JL, Fromy B. Cellular mechanisms underlying cutaneous pressure-induced vasodilation: in vivo involvement of potassium channels. Am J Physiol Heart Circ Physiol 289: H174-H180, 2005.

Gearing, A. J. and W. Newman (1993). "Circulating adhesion molecules in disease." Immunol Today 14(10): 506-12.

Giombini, A., Giovannini, V., Cesare, A. D., Pacetti, P., Ichinoseki-Sekine, N., Shiraishi, M., et al. (2007). Hyperthermia induced by microwave diathermy in the management of muscle and tendon injuries. *British Medical Bulletin 83*, 379-96.

Giordano, F. J. (2005). "Oxygen, oxidative stress, hypoxia, and heart failure." J Clin Invest 115(3): 500-8.

Goyal, H. O., T. D. Braden, et al. (2007). "Role of estrogen in induction of penile dysmorphogenesis: a review." Reproduction 134(2): 199-208.

Grana, W. A. (1993). Physical agents in musculoskeletal problems: heat and cold therapy modalities. Instr Course Lect, 42, 439-442.

Green, S., P. Walter, et al. (1986). "Cloning of the human oestrogen receptor cDNA." J Steroid Biochem 24(1): 77-83.

Gribbin B, Pickering TG, Sleight P: Effect of age and high blood pressure on baroreflex sensitivity in man. Circ Res, 1971; 29:424-431.

Grice, E. A., & Segre, J. A. (2011). The skin microbiome. Nat Rev Microbiol, 9(4), 244-253. doi:10.1038/nrmicro2537.

Griendling, K. K. and G. A. FitzGerald (2003a). "Oxidative stress and cardiovascular injury: Part I: basic mechanisms and in vivo monitoring of ROS." Circulation 108(16): 1912-6.

Griendling, K. K. and G. A. FitzGerald (2003b). "Oxidative stress and cardiovascular injury: Part II: animal and human studies." Circulation 108(17): 2034-40.

Griffin, M. E., M. J. Marcucci, et al. (1999). "Free fatty acid-induced insulin resistance is associated with activation of protein kinase C theta and alterations in the insulin signaling cascade." Diabetes 48(6): 1270-4.

Griffiths, C. E. M., Barker, J., Bleiker, T., Chalmers, R., & Creamer, D. (2016). Rook's textbook of dermatology (Ninth edition. ed.). Chichester, West Sussex ; Hoboken, NJ: John Wiley & Sons Inc.

Guo, X., Razandi, M., Pedram, A., Kassab, G., & Levin, E. (2005). Estrogen induces vascular wall dilation: mediation through kinase signaling to nitric oxide and estrogen receptors alpha & beta. The Journal of Biological chemistry, 280, 19704-19710.

Gupta, P. K., J. Subramani, et al. (2008). "Role of voltage-dependent potassium channels and myo-endothelial gap junctions in 4-aminopyridine-induced inhibition of acetylcholine relaxation in rat carotid artery." Eur J Pharmacol 591(1-3): 171-6.

Guyton, A. C. (2008). Textbook of Medical Physiology (11th Ed.): Elsevier Saunders.

Guyton S, Harris J: Pressoreceptor-autonomic oscillation: A probable cause of vasomotor waves. Am J Physiol, 1951; 165:158-166.

Haendeler J: Nitric oxide and endothelial cell aging. Eur J ClinPharmacol, 2006; 13: 137–40

Hafezi-Moghadam, A., T. Simoncini, et al. (2002). "Acute cardiovascular protective effects of corticosteroids are mediated by non-transcriptional activation of endothelial nitric oxide synthase." Nat Med 8(5): 473-9.

Hajjar, I. and T. A. Kotchen (2003). "Trends in prevalence, awareness, treatment, and control of hypertension in the United States, 1988-2000." JAMA 290(2): 199-206.

Hak, A. E., C. D. Stehouwer, et al. (1999). "Associations of C-reactive protein with measures of obesity, insulin resistance, and subclinical atherosclerosis in healthy, middle-aged women." Arterioscler Thromb Vasc Biol 19(8): 1986-91.

Hamada, H., M. K. Kim, et al. (2006). "Estrogen receptors alpha and beta mediate contribution of bone marrow-derived endothelial progenitor cells to functional recovery after myocardial infarction." Circulation 114(21): 2261-70.

Hanson GK,Janasson L,Seiffert PS. Immune mechanisms in atherosclerosis.Atherosclerosis 1989;9:567-8.

Hara K, Kubota N, Tobe K, Terauchi Y, Miki H, Komeda K, et al. The role of PPAR γ as a thrifty gene both in mice and humans. Br J Nutr 2002;84:S235-9.

Hare, J. M. (2004). "Nitroso-redox balance in the cardiovascular system." N Engl J Med 351(20): 2112-4.

Harris, G. (2005). Progress in medical ultrasound exposimetry. *IEEE Trans Ultrason Ferroelec Freq Contr. 52*, 717–736.

Harris, M. B., H. Ju, et al. (2001). "Reciprocal phosphorylation and regulation of endothelial nitric-oxide synthase in response to bradykinin stimulation." J Biol Chem 276(19): 16587-91.

Hashim, M. A. and A. S. Tadepalli (1995). "Cutaneous vasomotor effects of neuropeptide Y." Neuropeptides 29(5): 263-71.

Hawkes, A., Draper, D., Johnson, A., Diede, M., & Rigby, J. (2013). Heating capacity of ReBound shortwave diathermy and moist hot packs at superficial depths. *J Athl Train. 48(4)*, 471-476 .

Haynes, M. P., K. S. Russell, et al. (2000). "Molecular mechanisms of estrogen actions on the vasculature." J Nucl Cardiol 7(5): 500-8.

Heath, M. E. (1998). "Neuropeptide Y and Y1-receptor agonists increase blood flow through arteriovenous anastomoses in rat tail." J Appl Physiol 85(1): 301-9.

Heinrich, P. C., J. V. Castell, et al. (1990). "Interleukin-6 and the acute phase response." Biochem J 265(3): 621-36.

Heissig, B., K. Hattori, et al. (2002). "Recruitment of stem and progenitor cells from the bone marrow niche requires MMP-9 mediated release of kit-ligand." Cell 109(5): 625-37.

Hendee, W. (2013). Physics of Thermal Therapy: Fundamentals and Clinical Applications. Florida: Taylor & Francis.

Hisamoto, K., M. Ohmichi, et al. (2001). "Estrogen induces the Akt-dependent activation of endothelial nitric-oxide synthase in vascular endothelial cells." J Biol Chem 276(5): 3459-67.

Holowatz LA, Houghton BL, Wong BJ et al: Nitric oxide and attenuated refl ex cutaneous vasodilation in aged skin. Am J Physiol Heart CircPhysiol, 2003; 284: H1662–67

Hori, S. (1995). Adaptation to heat. Japanese journal of physiology, 45, 921-946.

Hotamisligil GS, Murray DL, Choy LN, Spiegelman BM. Tumor necrosis factr-α inhibits signaling from the insulin receptor. Proc Natl Acad Sci USA 1994;91:4854-8.

Houghton PE, N. E., Hoens AM. (2010). ELECTROPHYSICAL AGENTS - Contraindications And Precautions: An Evidence-Based Approach To Clinical Decision Making In Physical Therapy. Physiother Can, 62(5), 1-80. doi:10.3138/ptc.62.5

Houglum, P. A. (2016). Therapeutic Exercise for Musculoskeletal Injuries (4th ed.): Human Kinetics.

Hsueh WA, Law RD: Cardiovascular risk continuum: implications of insulin resistance and diabetes. Am J Med, 1998; 105(1A):4S-14S.

Hume, L., G. D. Oakley, et al. (1986). "Asymptomatic myocardial ischemia in diabetes and its relationship to diabetic neuropathy: an exercise electrocardiography study in middle-aged diabetic men." Diabetes Care 9(4): 384-8.

Hwang, S. J., C. M. Ballantyne, et al. (1997). "Circulating adhesion molecules VCAM-1, ICAM-1, and E-selectin in carotid atherosclerosis and incident coronary heart disease cases: the Atherosclerosis Risk In Communities (ARIC) study." Circulation 96(12): 4219-25.

Iafrati, M. D., R. H. Karas, et al. (1997). "Estrogen inhibits the vascular injury response in estrogen receptor alpha-deficient mice." Nat Med 3(5): 545-8.

Ignarro LJ,Buga GM,Wood KS,Byrns RE,Chaudhuri G,Endothelium-derived relaxing factor produced and released from artery and vein is nitric oxide.proc Natl Acad SciUSA 1987;84:9265-9269.(pubMed:2827174).

Itoh, N., K. Obata, et al. (1983). "Human preprovasoactive intestinal polypeptide contains a novel PHI-27-like peptide, PHM-27." Nature 304(5926): 547-9.

Iwakura, A., C. Luedemann, et al. (2003). "Estrogen-mediated, endothelial nitric oxide synthase-dependent mobilization of bone marrow-derived endothelial progenitor cells contributes to reendothelialization after arterial injury." Circulation 108(25): 3115-21.

Jager A, van Hinsberg VWM, Kostense PJ, Emeis JJ, Yudkin JS, Nijpels G, Dekker JM, Heine RJ, Bouter LM, Stehouwer CDA. Von Willebrand factor, C-reactive protein, and 5-year mortality in diabetic and non-diabetic subjects: The Hoorn study.Arterioscler Thromb vasc Biol 1999;19:3071-8.

Jager A, van Hinsberg VWN, Kostense PJ, Emeis JJ, Nijpels G, Dekker JM, Heine RJ,Bouter LM, Stehouwer CDA. Increased levels of soluble vascular adhesion molecule 1 are associated with risk of cardiovascular mortality in type 2 diabetes: The Hoorn study. Diabetes 2000;49:485-91.

Jain, T. K., & Sharma, N. K. (2014). The effectiveness of physiotherapeutic interventions in treatment of frozen shoulder/adhesive capsulitis: a systematic review. J Back Musculoskelet Rehabil, 27(3), 247-273. doi:10.3233/BMR-130443.

Jennings BL, Donald JA. Neurally-derived nitric oxide regulates vascular tone in pulmonary and cutaneous arteries of the toad, Bufo marinus. Am J Physiol Regul Integr Comp Physiol. 2008 Nov;295(5):R1640-6.

Jewo, P. I., & Fadeyibi, I. O. (2015). Progress in burns research: a review of advances in burn pathophysiology. Ann Burns Fire Disasters, 28(2), 105-115.

Johnson, J. M. (1986a). "Nonthermoregulatory control of human skin blood flow." J Appl Physiol 61(5): 1613-22.

Johnson, J. M., G. L. Brengelmann, et al. (1986b). "Regulation of the cutaneous circulation." Fed Proc 45(13): 2841-50.

Kagawa, Y., Y. Yanagisawa, et al. (2002). "Single nucleotide polymorphisms of thrifty genes for energy metabolism: evolutionary origins and prospects for intervention to prevent obesity-related diseases." Biochem Biophys Res Commun 295(2): 207-22.

Kahn, D. F., S. J. Duffy, et al. (2002). "Effects of black race on forearm resistance vessel function." Hypertension 40(2): 195-201.

Kalinowski, L., I. T. Dobrucki, et al. (2002). "Cerivastatin potentiates nitric oxide release and enos expression through inhibition of isoprenoids synthesis." J Physiol Pharmacol 53(4 Pt 1): 585-95.

Kalinowski, L., I. T. Dobrucki, et al. (2004). "Race-specific differences in endothelial function: predisposition of African Americans to vascular diseases." Circulation 109(21): 2511-7.

Kalra, L., C. Rambaran, et al. (2005). "Ethnic differences in arterial responses and inflammatory markers in Afro-Caribbean and Caucasian subjects." Arterioscler Thromb Vasc Biol 25(11): 2362-7.

Kamijo, Y., K. Lee, et al. (2005). "Active cutaneous vasodilation in resting humans during mild heat stress." J Appl Physiol 98(3): 829-37.

Karakitsos, D., A. P. Patrianakos, et al. (2006). "Androgen deficiency and endothelial dysfunction in men with end-stage kidney disease receiving maintenance hemodialysis." Am J Nephrol 26(6): 536-43.

Kato, N., T. Sugiyama, et al. (1999). "Lack of evidence for association between the endothelial nitric oxide synthase gene and hypertension." Hypertension 33(4): 933-6.

Kawashima S,Yokoyama M.Dysfunction of endothelial nitric oxide synthase and atherosclerosis.Arterioscler Thromb Vasc Biol 2004;24:998-1005.(pubMed; 15001455)

Keeble JE,Moore PK,Pharmacology and potential therapeutic applications of nitric oxide-releasing non-steroidal anti-inflammatory and related nitric oxide-donating drugs.Br J Pharmacol 2002;137:295-310.(pubMed: 12237248)

Kaltenborn, F. (2002). *Manual Mobilization of the Joints.* Minneapolis, MN.: OTPT.

Kellogg, D. L., Jr., C. G. Crandall, et al. (1998). "Nitric oxide and cutaneous active vasodilation during heat stress in humans." J Appl Physiol 85(3): 824-9.

Kellogg, D. L., Jr., G. J. Hodges, et al. (2007). "Cholinergic mechanisms of cutaneous active vasodilation during heat stress in cystic fibrosis." J Appl Physiol 103(3): 963-8.

Kellogg, D. L., Jr., J. L. Zhao, et al. (2003). "Nitric oxide concentration increases in the cutaneous interstitial space during heat stress in humans." J Appl Physiol 94(5): 1971-7.

Kellogg, D. L., Jr., J. M. Johnson, et al. (1989). "Selective abolition of adrenergic vasoconstrictor responses in skin by local iontophoresis of bretylium." Am J Physiol 257(5 Pt 2): H1599-606.

Kellogg, D. L., Jr., P. E. Pergola, et al. (1995). "Cutaneous active vasodilation in humans is mediated by cholinergic nerve cotransmission." Circ Res 77(6): 1222-8.

Kemmet, D. (1989). Premenstrual exacerbation of atopic dermatitis. British Journal of Dermatology, 120, 715-722.

Kenney, W. L., A. L. Morgan, et al. (1997). "Decreased active vasodilator sensitivity in aged skin." Am J Physiol 272(4 Pt 2): H1609-14.

Kim, K., R. J. Valentine, et al. (2008). "Associations of visceral adiposity and exercise participation with C-reactive protein, insulin resistance, and endothelial dysfunction in Korean healthy adults." Metabolism 57(9): 1181-9.

Kloth, L. C. (1995). Physical modalities in wound management: UVC, therapeutic heating and electrical stimulation. Ostomy Wound Manage, 41(5), 18-20, 22-14, 26-17.

Knight, K., Knight, K. L., & Draper, D. O. (2012). Therapeutic Modalities: The Art and Science. Philadelphia: Lippincott Williams & Wilkins.

Koeda, T., R. Tamura, et al. (2007). "Substance P is involved in the cutaneous blood flow increase response to sympathetic nerve stimulation in persistently inflamed rats." J Physiol Sci 57(6): 361-6.

Koldas Dogan, S., Sonel Tur, B., Kurtais, Y., & Atay, M. B. (2008). Comparison of three different approaches in the treatment of chronic low back pain. Clin Rheumatol, 27(7), 873-881. doi:10.1007/s10067-007-0815-7

Kone, B. C. (2000). "Protein-protein interactions controlling nitric oxide synthases." Acta Physiol Scand 168(1): 27-31.

Konrady AO, Rudomanov OG, Yacovleva OI, Shlyakhto EV: Power spectral components of heart rate variability in different types of cardiac remodelling in hypertensive patients. Med Sci Monit, 2001; 7(1):58-63.

Kosecik, M., O. Erel, et al. (2005). "Increased oxidative stress in children exposed to passive smoking." Int J Cardiol 100(1): 61-4.

Kozak, A. J., F. Liu, et al. (2005). "Role of peroxynitrite in the process of vascular tone regulation by nitric oxide and prostanoids--a nanotechnological approach." Prostaglandins Leukot Essent Fatty Acids 72(2): 105-13.

Krakoff, J., T. Funahashi, et al. (2003). "Inflammatory markers, adiponectin, and risk of type 2 diabetes in the Pima Indian." Diabetes Care 26(6): 1745-51.

Kravitz, C. A. V. a. L. (2004). Staying Cool When Your Body is Hot. Aquatic Exercise Association Journal(January), 16-17.

Kubes, P., Suzuki, M.,Granger, DN.Nitric oxide: an endogenous modulator of leukocyte adhesion.proc Natl Acad Sci USA 1991;88:4651-4655.(pubMed: 1675786)

Kuiper, G. G., E. Enmark, et al. (1996). "Cloning of a novel receptor expressed in rat prostate and ovary." Proc Natl Acad Sci U S A 93(12): 5925-30.

Kvandal P, Stefanovska A, Veber M, Kvernmo HD, Kirkeboen KA. Regulation of human cutaneous cirvulation evaluated by laser Doppler flowmetry, iontophoresis, and spectral analysis: importance of nitric oxide and prostaglandins. Microvasc Res. 2003 May;65(3):160-71.

Lacigova, S., L. Bartunek, et al. (2009). "Influence of cardiovascular autonomic neuropathy on atherogenesis and heart function in patients with type 1 diabetes." Diabetes Res Clin Pract 83(1): 26-31.

Lahm, T., K. M. Patel, et al. (2007). "Endogenous estrogen attenuates pulmonary artery vasoreactivity and acute hypoxic pulmonary vasoconstriction: the effects of sex and menstrual cycle." Am J Physiol Endocrinol Metab 293(3): E865-71.

Lahm, T., P. R. Crisostomo, et al. (2008). "The effects of estrogen on pulmonary artery vasoreactivity and hypoxic pulmonary vasoconstriction: potential new clinical implications for an old hormone." Crit Care Med 36(7): 2174-83.

Lam, T. H., Y. He, et al. (1997). "Mortality attributable to cigarette smoking in China." JAMA 278(18): 1505-8.

Lam, F. Y. and W. R. Ferrell (1993). "Acute inflammation in the rat knee joint attenuates sympathetic vasoconstriction but enhances neuropeptide-mediated vasodilatation assessed by laser Doppler perfusion imaging." Neuroscience 52(2): 443-9.

Lam, T. H., L. J. Liu, et al. (1999). "The relationship between fibrinogen and other coronary heart disease risk factors in a Chinese population." Atherosclerosis 143(2): 405-13.

Lammertink, B. H., Bos, C., Deckers, R., Storm, G., Moonen, C. T., & Escoffre, J. M. (2015). Sonochemotherapy: from bench to bedside. Front Pharmacol, 6, 138. doi:10.3389/fphar.2015.00138.

Langer, A., M. R. Freeman, et al. (1991). "Detection of silent myocardial ischemia in diabetes mellitus." Am J Cardiol 67(13): 1073-8.

Lapu-Bula, R. and E. Ofili (2007). "From hypertension to heart failure: role of nitric oxide-mediated endothelial dysfunction and emerging insights from myocardial contrast echocardiography." Am J Cardiol 99(6B): 7D-14D.

Lawson, D. and J. S. Petrofsky (2007). "A randomized control study on the effect of biphasic electrical stimulation in a warm room on skin blood flow and healing rates in chronic wounds of patients with and without diabetes." Med Sci Monit 13(6): CR258-63.

Lee SJ, Lee DW, Kim KS, Lee IK. (2001). "Effect of estrogen on endothelial dysfunction in postmenopausal women with diabetes. Diab Res and Clin Prac 54(2); s81-s92.

Leitgeb, N., Omerspahic, A., & Niedermayr, F. (2010). Exposure of non-target tissues in medical diathermy. *Bioelectromagnetics 31(1)*, 1-29.

Lenasi, H. and M. Strucl (2008). "The effect of nitric oxide synthase and cyclooxygenase inhibition on cutaneous microvascular reactivity." Eur J Appl Physiol 103(6): 719-26

Lewin, G. R. and L. M. Mendell (1993). "Nerve growth factor and nociception." Trends Neurosci 16(9): 353-9.

Lewis Jr., G. K., Olbricht, W. L., & Lewis, G. (2008). Acoustic enhanced Evans blue dye perfusion in neurological tissues. *Proceedings of Meetings on Acoustics 2 (1)*.

Li R, Ning Z, Cui J, Khalsa B, Ai L, Takabe W, Beebe T, Majumdar R, Sioutas C, Hsiai T, Li. Ultrafine particles from diesel engines induce vascular oxidative stress via JNK activation. Free Radic Biol Med. 2008 Dec 11.

Lloyd et al (2000), Does angina vary with menstrual cycle in women with pre-menopausal coronary artery disease? Heart, 84, 189-192

Lohman, E. B., 3rd, Bains, G. S., Lohman, T., DeLeon, M., & Petrofsky, J. S. (2011). A comparison of the effect of a variety of thermal and vibratory modalities on skin temperature and blood flow in healthy volunteers. Med Sci Monit, 17(9), MT72-81.

Lteif, A. A., K. Han, et al. (2005). "Obesity, insulin resistance, and the metabolic syndrome: determinants of endothelial dysfunction in whites and blacks." Circulation 112(1): 32-8.

Maiorana, A., G. O'Driscoll, et al. (2003). "Exercise and the nitric oxide vasodilator system." Sports Med 33(14): 1013-35.

Maloney-Hinds, C., J. S. Petrofsky, et al. (2008). "The effect of 30 Hz vs. 50 Hz passive vibration and duration of vibration on skin blood flow in the arm." Med Sci Monit 14(3): CR112-6.

Maloney-Hinds C, Petrofsky JS, Zimmerman G, Hessinger DA. The role of nitric oxide in skin blood flow increases due to vibration in healthy adults and adults with type 2 diabetes. Diabetes Technol Ther. 2009 Feb; 11(1): 39-43

Martin, H. L., J. L. Loomis, et al. (1995). "Maximal skin vascular conductance in subjects aged 5-85 yr." J Appl Physiol 79(1): 297-301.

Masiero, S. (2008). Thermal rehabilitation and osteoarticular diseases of the elderly. Aging Clin Exp Res, 20(3), 189-194.

Mason, R. P., L. Kalinowski, et al. (2005). "Nebivolol reduces nitroxidative stress and restores nitric oxide bioavailability in endothelium of black Americans." Circulation 112(24): 3795-801.

Mata-Greenwood E, Chen DB. 2008. "Racial differences in Nitic Oxide-Dependent Vasorelaxation. Reprod Sci January;15(1):9-25.

Mates, J. M. (2000). "Effects of antioxidant enzymes in the molecular control of reactive oxygen species toxicology." Toxicology 153(1-3): 83-104.

Mayer, J. M., Ralph, L., Look, M., Erasala, G. N., Verna, J. L., Matheson, L. N., & Mooney, V. (2005). Treating acute low back pain with continuous low-level heat wrap therapy and/or exercise: a randomized controlled trial. Spine J, 5(4), 395-403. doi:10.1016/j.spinee.2005.03.009

McDougall, J. J., S. M. Karimian, et al. (1994). "Alteration of substance P-mediated vasodilatation and sympathetic vasoconstriction in the rat knee joint by adjuvant-induced inflammation." Neurosci Lett 174(2): 127-9.

McDougall, J. J., S. M. Karimian, et al. (1995). "Prolonged alteration of vasoconstrictor and vasodilator responses in rat knee joints by adjuvant monoarthritis." Exp Physiol 80(3): 349-57.

McBean, A. M., S. Li, et al. (2004). "Differences in diabetes prevalence, incidence, and mortality among the elderly of four racial/ethnic groups: whites, blacks, hispanics, and asians." Diabetes Care 27(10): 2317-24.

McCulloch, J. (1995). Physical modalities in wound management: ultrasound, vasopneumatic devices and hydrotherapy. Ostomy Wound Manage, 41(5), 30-32, 34, 36-37.

McDaniel, M., C. Paxson, et al. (2006). "Racial disparities in childhood asthma in the United States: evidence from the National Health Interview Survey, 1997 to 2003." Pediatrics 117(5): e868-77.

McKeigue, P. M., B. Shah, et al. (1991). "Relation of central obesity and insulin resistance with high diabetes prevalence and cardiovascular risk in South Asians." Lancet 337(8738): 382-6.

McLaughlin, V. V. and M. D. McGoon (2006). "Pulmonary arterial hypertension." Circulation 114(13): 1417-31.

McLellan, K., J. S. Petrofsky, et al. (2008). "The effects of skin moisture and subcutaneous fat thickness on the ability of the skin to dissipate heat in young and old subjects, with and without diabetes, at three environmental room temperatures." Med Eng Phys.

Michell, B. J., J. E. Griffiths, et al. (1999). "The Akt kinase signals directly to endothelial nitric oxide synthase." Curr Biol 9(15): 845-8

Michlovitz, S. L., Bellew, J. W., & Jr, T. P. (2011). *Modalities for Therapeutic Intervention.* F.A. Davis.

Miwa, K., M. Fujita, et al. (2005). "Recent insights into the mechanisms, predisposing factors, and racial differences of coronary vasospasm." Heart Vessels 20(1): 1-7.

Mo, S., Coussios, C.-C., Seymour, L., & Carlisle, R. (2012). Ultrasound-Enhanced Drug Delivery for Cancer. *Expert Opinion on Drug Delivery 9 (12)*, 1525.

Montagnani, M., H. Chen, et al. (2001). "Insulin-stimulated activation of eNOS is independent of Ca2+ but requires phosphorylation by Akt at Ser(1179)." J Biol Chem 276(32): 30392-8.

Montain SJ, Coyle EF: Fluid ingestion during exercise skin blood flow independent of increases in blood volume. J Appl Physiol, 1992;73(3):903-10.

Morris, J. L. (1999). "Cotransmission from sympathetic vasoconstrictor neurons to small cutaneous arteries in vivo." Am J Physiol 277(1 Pt 2): H58-64.

Mount, P. F., B. E. Kemp, et al. (2007). "Regulation of endothelial and myocardial NO synthesis by multi-site eNOS phosphorylation." J Mol Cell Cardiol 42(2): 271-9.

Mowa, CN., Hoch, R., Montavon, CL., Jesmin, S., Hindman, G., Hou, G. (2008) Biomedical Research 29(5)267-270.

Mun, J. H., Jeon, J. H., Jung, Y. J., Jang, K. U., Yang, H. T., Lim, H. J., . . . Seo, C. H. (2012). The factors associated with contact burns from therapeutic modalities. Ann Rehabil Med, 36(5), 688-695. doi:10.5535/arm.2012.36.5.688

Murphy, C., G. S. Kanaganayagam, et al. (2007). "Vascular dysfunction and reduced circulating endothelial progenitor cells in young healthy UK South Asian men." Arterioscler Thromb Vasc Biol 27(4): 936-42.

Murray, D. P., T. O'Brien, et al. (1990). "Autonomic dysfunction and silent myocardial ischaemia on exercise testing in diabetes mellitus." Diabet Med 7(7): 580-4.

Nadler, S. F., Weingand, K., & Kruse, R. J. (2004). The Physiologic Basis and Clinical Applications of Cryotherapy and Thermotherapy for the Pain Practitioner. *Pain Physician. 7*, 395-399.

Nappo, F., K. Esposito, et al. (2002). "Postprandial endothelial activation in healthy subjects and in type 2 diabetic patients: role of fat and carbohydrate meals." J Am Coll Cardiol 39(7): 1145-50.

Narkiewicz, K., P. J. van de Borne, et al. (1998). "Cigarette smoking increases sympathetic outflow in humans." Circulation 98(6): 528-34.

Niakan, E., Y. Harati, et al. (1986). "Silent myocardial infarction and diabetic cardiovascular autonomic neuropathy." Arch Intern Med 146(11): 2229-30.

Nicol, N. H. (2005). Anatomy and physiology of the skin. Dermatol Nurs, 17(1), 62.

Nilsson, T., D. Erlinge, et al. (1996). "Contractile effects of neuropeptide Y in human subcutaneous resistance arteries are mediated by Y1 receptors." J Cardiovasc Pharmacol 28(6): 764-8.

Nissen, N. N., P. J. Polverini, et al. (1998). "Vascular endothelial growth factor mediates angiogenic activity during the proliferative phase of wound healing." Am J Pathol 152(6): 1445-52.

Northam, E. A., D. Rankins, et al. (2009). "Central nervous system function in youth with type 1 diabetes 12 years after disease onset." Diabetes Care.

Novello, A. C. (1990). "Surgeon General's report on the health benefits of smoking cessation." Public Health Rep 105(6): 545-8.

O'Brien, K. D., T. O. McDonald, et al. (1996). "Neovascular expression of E-selectin, intercellular adhesion molecule-1, and vascular cell adhesion molecule-1 in human atherosclerosis and their relation to intimal leukocyte content." Circulation 93(4): 672-82.

O'Toole TE, Conklin DJ, Bhatnagar A. Environmental risk factors for heart disease. Rev Environ Health. 2008 Jul-Sep;23(3):167-202.

Page, M. J., Green, S., Kramer, S., Johnston, R. V., McBain, B., & Buchbinder, R. (2014). Electrotherapy modalities for adhesive capsulitis (frozen shoulder). Cochrane Database Syst Rev(10), CD011324. doi:10.1002/14651858.CD011324

Parsons, K. (2009). Maintaining health, comfort and productivity in heat waves. Glob Health Action, 2. doi:10.3402/gha.v2i0.2057.

Pare, G., A. Krust, et al. (2002). "Estrogen receptor-alpha mediates the protective effects of estrogen against vascular injury." Circ Res 90(10): 1087-92.

Patterson, G. C. (1956). "The role of intravascular pressure in the causation of reactive hyperaemia in the human forearm." Clin Sci (Lond) 15(1): 17-25.

Periaswamy, R., U. Gurusamy, et al. (2008). "Gender specific association of endothelial nitric oxide synthase gene (Glu298Asp) polymorphism with essential hypertension in a south Indian population." Clin Chim Acta 395(1-2): 134-6.

Peter, R., O. E. Okoseime, et al. (2009). "Postprandial glucose - a potential therapeutic target to reduce cardiovascular mortality." Curr Vasc Pharmacol 7(1): 68-74.

Petrofsky J., LeDonne, D., Rineheart, J. & Linda, A (1976) Isometric strength and endurance during the menstrual cycle. European journal of applied physiology, 35, 1-10.

Petrofsky JS, Besonis C, Rivera D, Schwab E, Lee S: Does Local Heating Really Help Diabetic Patients Increase Circulation. J Orthop Neurol Surg, 2003a; 21:40-48.

Petrofsky JS, Besonis C, Rivera D, Schwab E, Lee S: Heat Tolerance in patients with diabetes. J Appl Research, 2003b; 3:28-34.

Petrofsky, J.S., Bweir, S., Lee, S., & Libarona, M. (2004). Rosiglitazone Improves Age Related Reductions in Forearm Resting Flows and Endothelial Dysfunction Observed in Type 2 Diabetes. Diabetes, 53;A141.

Petrofsky J, Lee S. The effects of type 2 diabetes and aging on vascular endothelial and autonomic function. Med Sci Monit. 2005a Jun;11(6):CR247-254.

Petrofsky J, Lee S, Cuneo M. Effects of aging and type 2 diabetes on resting and post occlusive hyperemia of the forearm; the impact of rosiglitazone. BMC Endocr Disord. 2005b Mar 24;5(1):4.

Petrofsky, J. S., E. Lohman, 3rd, et al. (2006a). "The influence of alterations in room temperature on skin blood flow during contrast baths in patients with diabetes." Med Sci Monit 12(7): CR290-5.

Petrofsky, J.S., Lohman, E. III,Suh, H.J., Garcia, J., Anders, A., Sutterfield, C., Khandge, C. The effect of aging on conductive heat exchange in the skin at two environmental temperatures. Med Sci Monit. 2006b Oct;12(10):CR400-8.

Petrofsky, J., A. Al Malty, et al. (2007a). "Isometric endurance, body and skin temperature and limb and skin blood flow during the menstrual cycle." Med Sci Monit 13(3): CR111-7.

Petrofsky, J., Bains, G., Prowse, M., Gunda, S., Berk, L., Raju, C., . . . Madani, P. (2009). Dry heat, moist heat and body fat: are heating modalities really effective in people who are overweight? J Med Eng Technol, 33(5), 361-369. doi:10.1080/03091900802355508.

Petrofsky, J., Berk, L., Bains, G., Khowailed, I. A., Hui, T., Granado, M., . . . Lee, H. (2013). Moist heat or dry heat for delayed onset muscle soreness. J Clin Med Res, 5(6), 416-425. doi:10.4021/jocmr1521w.

Petrofsky, J., C. M. Hinds, et al. (2007b). "The interrelationships between electrical stimulation, the environment surrounding the vascular endothelial cells of the skin, and the role of nitric oxide in mediating the blood flow response to electrical stimulation." Med Sci Monit 13(9): CR391-397.

Petrofsky J, Hinds CM, Batt J, Prowse M, Suh HJ.The interrelationships between electrical stimulation, the environment surrounding the vascular endothelial cells of the skin, and the role of nitric oxide in mediating the blood flow response to electrical stimulation. Med Sci Monit. 2007c Sep;13(9):CR391-397.

Petrofsky, J. S., D. Lawson, et al. (2007d). "The influence of local versus global heat on the healing of chronic wounds in patients with diabetes." Diabetes Technol Ther 9: 535-44.

Petrofsky, J. S., & Laymon, M. (2009). Heat transfer to deep tissue: the effect of body fat and heating modality. J Med Eng Technol, 33(5), 337-348. doi:10.1080/03091900802069547

Petrofsky, J., S. Lee, et al. (2007e). "The effect of rosiglitazone on orthostatic tolerance during heat exposure in individuals with type II diabetes." Diabetes Technol Ther 9: 377-86.

Petrofsky, J., E. Lohman, 3rd, et al. (2007f). "Effects of contrast baths on skin blood flow on the dorsal and plantar foot in people with type 2 diabetes and age-matched controls." Physiother Theory Pract 23: 189-97.

Petrofsky JS, AlMalty A, Prowse M. Relationship between multiple stimuli and skin blood flow. 2008a. Med Sci Moni 14:CR399-405.

Petrofsky, JS, Bains, G., Chinna, R., Lohman, E., Berk, L., Prowse, M., Gunda, S., Madani, P, Batt, J (2008b) Moist vrs Dry heat as determinates of the blood flow response of the skin. submitted Med Sci Monit.

Petrofsky, JS, Bains, G., Prowse, M., Gunda, S., Berk, L., Chinna, R., Ethiraju, G., Vanarasa, D., Madani, P (2008c) Does Skin Moisture Influence The Blood Flow Response To Local Heat? A reevaluation of the Pennes Model. Submitted J Med Eng Tech

Petrofsky, J. S., K. McLellan, et al. (2008d). "Skin heat dissipation: the influence of diabetes, skin thickness, and subcutaneous fat thickness." Diabetes Technol Ther 10(6): 487-93.

Petrofsky, J.S., Prowse, M., & Lohman , E. (2008e). The influence of aging and diabetes on skin and subcutaneous fat thickness in different regions of the body. J Appl Res Clin Exp Ther. 8;55-61.

Petrofsky, J.S., Raju, C., Bains, G., Bogseth, M., Focil, N., Sirichotiratana, M., Hashemi, V., Gunda, S., Vallabhaneni, P., Kim, Y., Madani, P., Coords, H., McClurg, M., Lohman, E. Impact of hydrotherapy on skin blood flow; how much is due to the moisture and how much is due to heat? 2008f in press Physiother. Theory and Practice.

Pickup, J.C., Mattock, M.B., Chusney, G.D., Burt, D. NIDDM as a disease of the innate immune system: association of acute phase reactants and interleukin-6 with metabolic syndrome X. Diabetologia 1997;40:1286-92.

Pickup, J. C. and M. A. Crook (1998). "Is type II diabetes mellitus a disease of the innate immune system?" Diabetologia 41(10): 1241-8.

Potenza, M. A., S. Gagliardi, et al. (2009). "Endothelial dysfunction in diabetes: from mechanisms to therapeutic targets." Curr Med Chem 16(1): 94-112.

Prentice, W. E., Quillen, W. S., & Underwood, F. B. (2005). *Therapeutic modalities in rehabilitation.* New York: McGraw-Hill.

Puig T, Marti B, Rickenbach M, Dai SF, Casacuberta C, Wietlisbach V, Gutzwiller F. Some determinants of body weight, subcutaneous fat, and fat distribution in 25-64 year old Swiss urban men and woman. Soz Praventivmed. 1990;35(6):193-200.

Rabini, A., Piazzini, D. B., Tancredi, G., Foti, C., Milano, G., Ronconi, G., . . . Marzetti, E. (2012). Deep heating therapy via microwave diathermy relieves pain and improves physical function in patients with knee osteoarthritis: a double-blind randomized clinical trial. Eur J Phys Rehabil Med, 48(4), 549-559.

Rabinovitch, M., W. J. Gamble, et al. (1981). "Age and sex influence on pulmonary hypertension of chronic hypoxia and on recovery." Am J Physiol 240(1): H62-72.

Radha, V., K. S. Vimaleswaran, et al. (2006). "Role of genetic polymorphism peroxisome proliferator-activated receptor-gamma2 Pro12Ala on ethnic susceptibility to diabetes in South-Asian and Caucasian subjects: Evidence for heterogeneity." Diabetes Care 29(5): 1046-51.

Radomski, M. W., R. M. Palmer, et al. (1987). "The role of nitric oxide and cGMP in platelet adhesion to vascular endothelium." Biochem Biophys Res Commun 148(3): 1482-9.

Rahman, I., S. K. Biswas, et al. (2006). "Oxidant and antioxidant balance in the airways and airway diseases." Eur J Pharmacol 533(1-3): 222-39.

Rand, S. E., Goerlich, C., Marchand, K., & Jablecki, N. (2007). The physical therapy prescription. Am Fam Physician, 76(11), 1661-1666.

Rauhala, P., Andoh, T.,Chiueh, C.C.Neuroprotective properties of nitric oxide and S nitrosoglutathione.Toxicol Appl Pharmacol 2005;207:91-95.(pubMed: 15987648).

Ray CA, Monahan KD: Aging attenuates the vestibulosympathetic reflex in humans. Circulation, 2002; 26:956-61.

Ricciardolo, F. L. (2003). "Multiple roles of nitric oxide in the airways." Thorax 58(2): 175-82.

Ridker, P. M., C. H. Hennekens, et al. (1998). "Plasma concentration of soluble intercellular adhesion molecule 1 and risks of future myocardial infarction in apparently healthy men." Lancet 351(9096): 88-92.

Robertson, V. J., & Baker, K. G. (2001). A Review of Therapeutic Ultrasound: Effectiveness Studies. *Physical Therapy 81 (7)*, 1339–50.

Roddie, I. C., J. T. Shepherd, et al. (1957). "The contribution of constrictor and dilator nerves to the skin vasodilatation during body heating." J Physiol 136(3): 489-97.

Romano, R. A., & Sinha, S. (2011). Dynamic life of a skin keratinocyte: an intimate tryst with the master regulator p63. Indian J Exp Biol, 49(10), 721-731.

Rowell, L. B. (1974). "Human cardiovascular adjustments to exercise and thermal stress." Physiol Rev 54(1): 75-159.

Rowell, L. B. (1977). "Reflex control of the cutaneous vasculature." J Invest Dermatol 69(1): 154-66.

Rzeczuch, K., Jagielski, D., Kolodziej, A., Kaczmarek, A., Mielnik, M., Banasiak, W., Ponikowski, P. Coronary collateral circulation is less developed when ischaemic heart disease coexists with diabetes. Kardiol Pol 2003, 58 (2):85-92. Sarrel, P. (1990). Ovarian hormones and the circulation. Maturias, 121, 287-298.

Sagliocco L, Sartucci F, Giampietro O, Murri L: Amplitude loss of electrically and magnetically evoked sympathetic skin responses in early stages of type 1 (insulin-dependent) diabetes mellitus without signs of dysautonomia. Clin Auton Res, 1999; 9:5-10.

Scherre, U.,Sartori, C.Defective nitric oxide synthesis: a link between metabolic insulin resistance,sympathetic overactivity and cardiovascular mobidity.Eur j Endocrinol 2000:142:315-323.9 pubMed:10754469).

Schutzer, W.E., Mader, S.L. Age-related changes in vascular adrenergic signaling: clinical and mechanistic implications. Aging Res Rev 2003, 2(2):169-90.

Schwartz, R.S., Shuman, W.P., Bradbury, V.L., Cain, K.C., Fellingham, G.W., Beard, J.C., Kahn, S.E., Stratton, J.R., Cerqueira, M.D., Abrass, I.B. Body fat distribution in healthy young and older men. J Gerontol. 1990 Nov;45(6):M181-5.

Scremin, G., Kenney, W.L. Aging and the skin blood flow response to the unloading of baroreceptors during heat and cold stress. J Appl Physiol, 2004; 96(3):1019-25.

Sears, C.E.,Casadei, B. Mechanisms controlling blood flow and arterial pressure. Surgery 2002;20(3):i-v.

Shabana, Khan, S. S., Asmaa Alyaemni (2013). A Comparison of Superficial Heat, Deep Heat and Cold for Improving Plantar Flexors Extensibility. Middle-East Journal of Scientific Research, 13(4), 477-482. doi: 10.5829/idosi.mejsr.2013.13.4.72109.

Shakoor, M., Rahman, M., & Moyeenuzzaman, M. (2008). Effects of deep heat therapy on the patients with chronic low back pain. *Mymensingh Medical Journal 17(2)*, 32-8.

Shastry, S., N. M. Dietz, et al. (1998). "Effects of nitric oxide synthase inhibition on cutaneous vasodilation during body heating in humans." J Appl Physiol 85(3): 830-4.

Shi, Q., S. Rafii, et al. (1998). "Evidence for circulating bone marrow-derived endothelial cells." Blood 92(2): 362-7.

Shi, H.P., Efron, D.T., Most, D., Barbul, A. The role of iNOS in wound healing. Surgery, 2001; 130:225-229.

Shoji, M., S. Tsutaya, et al. (2000). "Positive association of endothelial nitric oxide synthase gene polymorphism with hypertension in northern Japan." Life Sci 66(26): 2557-62.

Siebert, J., Drabik, P., Lango, R., Szyndler, K. Stroke volume variability and heart rate power spectrum in relation to posture changes in healthy subjects. Med Sci Monit, 2004; 10(2):MT31-7.

Siguado-Roussel D, Demiot C, et al. Early endothelial dysfunction severely impairs skin blood flow response to local pressure application in streptozotocin-induced diabetic mice. Diabetes. 2004 Jun;53(6):1564-9.

Sokolnicki L, Khosla S, Charkoudian N. (2007) "Effects of testosterone and estradiol on cutaneous vasodilation during local warming in older men. Am J Physiol End Metab 293:E1426-E1429.

Sokolnicki, L. A., N. A. Strom, et al. (2008). "Skin blood flow and nitric oxide during body heating in type 2 diabetes mellitus." J Appl Physiol.

Srivastava, K., R. Narang, et al. (2008). "Association of eNOS Glu298Asp gene polymorphism with essential hypertension in Asian Indians." Clin Chim Acta 387(1-2): 80-3.

Stadler, K., Jenei, V., von Bolcshazy, G., Somogyi, A., Jakus, J. Increased nitric oxide levels as an early sign of premature aging in diabetes. Free Radic Biol Med 2003, 15 (35):1240-51.

Stansberry, K.B., Peppard, H.R., Babyak, L.M., Popp, G., McNitt, P.M., Vinik, Al.Primary nociceptive afferents mediate the blood flow dysfunction in non-glabrous (hairy) skin of type 2 diabetes: a new model for the pathogenesis of microvascular dysfunction. Diabetes Care, 1999; 22:1549-1554.

Starkey, C. (2013). *Therapeutic Modalities.* F.A. Davis.

Stephens, D. P., K. Aoki, et al. (2001). "Nonnoradrenergic mechanism of reflex cutaneous vasoconstriction in men." Am J Physiol Heart Circ Physiol 280(4): H1496-504.

Stephens, D. P., L. A. Bennett, et al. (2002). "Sympathetic nonnoradrenergic cutaneous vasoconstriction in women is associated with reproductive hormone status." Am J Physiol Heart Circ Physiol 282(1): H264-72.

Stephens, D. P., A. R. Saad, et al. (2004). "Neuropeptide Y antagonism reduces reflex cutaneous vasoconstriction in humans." Am J Physiol Heart Circ Physiol 287(3): H1404-9.

Stoll, A. M. (1977). THERMAL PROPERTIES OF HUMAN SKIN RELATED TO NONDESTRUCTUVE MEASUREMENT OF EPIDERMAL THICKNESS. Journal of Investigative Dermatology, 69(3), 328-332. doi:10.1111/1523-1747.ep12507865.

Strehlow, K., N. Werner, et al. (2003). "Estrogen increases bone marrow-derived endothelial progenitor cell production and diminishes neointima formation." Circulation 107(24): 3059-65.

Stuart-Smith K. Demystified: nitric oxide.Mol Pathol 2002;55:360-366 (PubMED:12456772)

Suh, H., Petrofsky JS., Fish, A. Hernandez, V., Mendoza, E., Collins, K., Yang, T., Abdul, A., Batt, J. (2008) A new electrode design to improve outcomes in the treatment of chronic non healing diabetic wounds. In press Diab Tech Ther.

Sun Q, Yue P, Deiuliis JA, Lumeng CN, Kampfrath T, Mikolaj MB, Cai Y, Ostrowski MC, Lu B, Parthasarathy S, Brook RD, Moffatt-Bruce SD, Chen LC, Rajagopalan S. Ambient air pollution exaggerates adipose inflammation and insulin resistance in a mouse model of diet-induced obesity. Circulation. 2009 Feb 3;119(4):538-46. Epub 2009 Jan 19.

Suri, J. S. (2008). *Advances in Diagnostic and Therapeutic Ultrasound Imaging.* Norwood: Artech House.

Tai, E. S., D. Corella, et al. (2004). "Differential effects of the C1431T and Pro12Ala PPARgamma gene variants on plasma lipids and diabetes risk in an Asian population." J Lipid Res 45(4): 674-85.

Taylor, W. F., S. E. DiCarlo, et al. (1992). "Neurogenic vasodilator control of rabbit ear blood flow." Am J Physiol 262(5 Pt 2): R766-70.

Taylor, W. F. and V. S. Bishop (1993). "A role for nitric oxide in active thermoregulatory vasodilation." Am J Physiol 264(5 Pt 2): H1355-9.

Thomas, G. N., P. Chook, et al. (2008). "Smoking without exception adversely affects vascular structure and function in apparently healthy Chinese: implications in global atherosclerosis prevention." Int J Cardiol 128(2): 172-7.

Thompson, C. S. and W. L. Kenney (2004). "Altered neurotransmitter control of reflex vasoconstriction in aged human skin." J Physiol 558(Pt 2): 697-704.

Triggle, C. R., M. Hollenberg, et al. (2003). "The endothelium in health and disease--a target for therapeutic intervention." J Smooth Muscle Res 39(6): 249-67.

Tripathy, D., P. Mohanty, et al. (2003). "Elevation of free fatty acids induces inflammation and impairs vascular reactivity in healthy subjects." Diabetes 52(12): 2882-7.

Tsai, W. C., Y. H. Li, et al. (2004). "Effects of oxidative stress on endothelial function after a high-fat meal." Clin Sci (Lond) 106(3): 315-9.

TUTEJA N, Chandra M,Tuteja R,Misra MK,Nitric oxide as a unique bioactive signaling messenger in physiology and pathophysiology.J Biomed Biotechnol 2004;2004;227-237.(pubMed 15467163).

Van der Poll T, Van Deventer SJH, Pasterkamp G,van Mourik JA, Buller HR,ten cate JW. Tumour necrosis factor induces von Willebrand factor release in healthy humans. Thromb Haemost 1992;67:623-6.

Vapaatalo, H. and E. Mervaala (2001). "Clinically important factors influencing endothelial function." Med Sci Monit 7(5): 1075-85.

Varsik P, Kucera P, Buranova D, Balaz M: Is the spinal cord lesion rare in diabetes mellitus? Somatosensory evoked potentials and central conduction time in diabetes mellitus. Med Sci Monit, 2001; 7(4):712-5.

Venkov, C. D., A. B. Rankin, et al. (1996). "Identification of authentic estrogen receptor in cultured endothelial cells. A potential mechanism for steroid hormone regulation of endothelial function." Circulation 94(4): 727-33.

Vinik, A. I., R. E. Maser, et al. (2003). "Diabetic autonomic neuropathy." Diabetes Care 26(5): 1553-79.

Walker, V. R. and K. S. Korach (2004). "Estrogen receptor knockout mice as a model for endocrine research." ILAR J 45(4): 455-61.

Wallenstein, S., C. L. Zucker, et al. (1980). "Some statistical methods useful in circulation research." Circ Res 47(1): 1-9.

Wang, S. Z., S. Z. Zhu, et al. (1994). "Efficient coupling of m5 muscarinic acetylcholine receptors to activation of nitric oxide synthase." J Pharmacol Exp Ther 268(2): 552-7.

Watanabe, H., K. Yamane, et al. (2004). "Influence of westernization of lifestyle on the progression of IMT in Japanese." J Atheroscler Thromb 11(6): 330-4.

Weyer, C., P. A. Tataranni, et al. (2000). "Insulin action and insulinemia are closely related to the fasting complement C3, but not acylation stimulating protein concentration." Diabetes Care 23(6): 779-85.

Weyer, C., J. S. Yudkin, et al. (2002). "Humoral markers of inflammation and endothelial dysfunction in relation to adiposity and in vivo insulin action in Pima Indians." Atherosclerosis 161(1): 233-42.

Wilkins, B. W., L. H. Chung, et al. (2004). "Mechanisms of vasoactive intestinal peptide-mediated vasodilation in human skin." J Appl Physiol 97(4): 1291-8.

Wilkins, B. W., B. J. Wong, et al. (2005). "Vasoactive intestinal peptide fragment VIP10-28 and active vasodilation in human skin." J Appl Physiol 99(6): 2294-301.

William E. Prentice, D. D. A. (2008). Arnheim's Principles of Athletic Training: A Competency-Based Approach with ESims (13 ed.). NY: McGraw-Hill Higher Education.

Winer N, Sowers JR: Vascular compliance in diabetes. Curr Diab Rep, 2003; 3(3):230-4.

Wong, B. J., B. W. Wilkins, et al. (2004). "H1 but not H2 histamine receptor activation contributes to the rise in skin blood flow during whole body heating in humans." J Physiol 560(Pt 3): 941-8.

Wong, R. A., Schumann, B., Townsend, R., & Phelps, C. A. (2007). A survey of therapeutic ultrasound use by physical therapists who are orthopaedic certified specialists. Phys Ther, 87(8), 986-994. doi:10.2522/ptj.20050392.

Woo, K. S., J. T. Robinson, et al. (1997). "Differences in the effect of cigarette smoking on endothelial function in chinese and white adults." Ann Intern Med 127(5): 372-5.

Woo, K. S., P. Chook, et al. (1999). "Westernization of Chinese adults and increased subclinical atherosclerosis." Arterioscler Thromb Vasc Biol 19(10): 2487-93.

Wyss, J., Patel, A. (2012). Therapeutic Programs for Musculoskeletal Disorders (1st ed.): Demos Medical.

Xu, F., Wen, T., Lu, T. J., & Seffen, K. A. (2008). Skin biothermomechanics for medical treatments. J Mech Behav Biomed Mater, 1(2), 172-187. doi:10.1016/j.jmbbm.2007.09.001.

Yildiriim, M. A., Ucar, D., & Ones, K. (2015). Comparison of therapeutic duration of therapeutic ultrasound in patients with knee osteoarthritis. J Phys Ther Sci, 27(12), 3667-3670. doi:10.1589/jpts.27.3667.

Yip, T.W.C.,Chook, P., Feng, X.H.,et al. Heavy passive smoking in casino is associated with higher atherosclerosis risk. Heart, Lung and Circulation 2007;24:739-43.

Yudkin, J. S., C. D. Stehouwer, et al. (1999). "C-reactive protein in healthy subjects: associations with obesity, insulin resistance, and endothelial dysfunction: a potential role for cytokines originating from adipose tissue?" Arterioscler Thromb Vasc Biol 19(4): 972-8.

Yudkin, J. S., M. Kumari, et al. (2000). "Inflammation, obesity, stress and coronary heart disease: is interleukin-6 the link?" Atherosclerosis 148(2): 209-14.

Yokota, T. and G. K. Hansson (1995). "Immunological mechanisms in atherosclerosis." J Intern Med 238(6): 479-89.

Zhou, Y. (2015). *Principles and Applications of Therapeutic Ultrasound in Healthcare.* Boca Raton: CRC Press.

Zhu, Y. J., & Lu, T. J. (2010). A multi-scale view of skin thermal pain: from nociception to pain sensation. Philos Trans A Math Phys Eng Sci, 368(1912), 521-559. doi:10.1098/rsta.2009.0234.

Zhu, Y., Z. Bian, et al. (2002). "Abnormal vascular function and hypertension in mice deficient in estrogen receptor beta." Science 295(5554): 505-8.

BLESSINGS

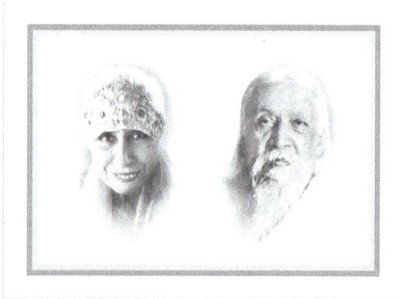

The Mother & Maharshi Aurobindo

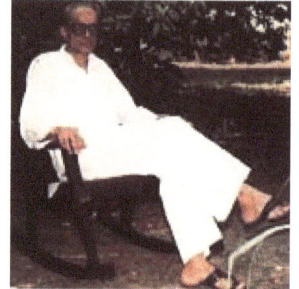

Dr. Ashwinbhai Kapadia

The very first publication of Dr. Bhargav Dave namely, "Heat and Human Interaction," is really, a boon from the divine mother to his scholastic study of human anatomy, and from the spiritual study of the energy in the form of heat, being generated and mobilize, throughout the different channels, physical, psychological, and psychic of the centrally located consciousness. It is really a De-Novo psychic science and it will lead the human world, to the next evolutionary mutation. It is really mother's blessings in the form of new conceptual reality, of tomorrow and of the spiritual age. I heartily congratulate Dr. Bhargav Dave for offering this psycho-spiritual treasure of knowledge, research and vision to the world. I pray to the divine mother to shower Her choicest blessing on him to enhance, his march and with the result to offer many such master pieces to the new human world of tomorrow.

Dr. Ashwinbhai Kapadia
Ex- Vice Chancellor,
South Gujarat University,
Surat, Gujarat, India
09-21-2016
Bhadrva-Vad-Pancham

Notes

www.ingramcontent.com/pod-product-compliance
Lightning Source LLC
Chambersburg PA
CBHW052051190326
41519CB00002BA/179